GUIDE TO TOTAL FITNESS OF BODY AND MIND

GUIDE TO TOTAL FITNESS OF BODY AND MIND

DR. R. KUMAR
MBBS, MS Ex-PGI

and

DR. MEENAL KUMAR
MBBS, MD, DGO

Preface by

DR. SUBHASH VARMA
Professor and Head,
Department of Internal Medicine,
PGI, Chandigarh

DEEP & DEEP PUBLICATIONS PVT. LTD.
F-159, Rajouri Garden, New Delhi-110027

GUIDE TO
TOTAL FITNESS OF BODY AND MIND

ISBN 81-7629-545-0

Typeset by S.S. COMPOSERS
3190, Mohindra Park, Shakur Basti, Delhi-110034.

Printed in India at ELEGANT PRINTERS,
A-38/2, Mayapuri Industrial Area, Phase-I, New Delhi-110 064.

Published by DEEP & DEEP PUBLICATIONS PVT. LTD.,
F-159, Rajouri Garden, New Delhi - 110 027
Phones : 25435369, 25440916
E-mails : deep98@del3.vsnl.net.in • ddpbooks@yahoo.co.in
Showroom :
2/13, Ansari Road, Daryaganj, New Delhi -110 002 • Telefax : 23245122

Contents

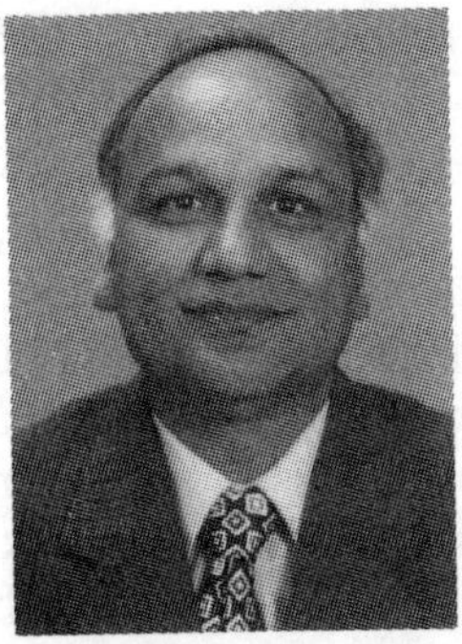

Preface

Human fitness and health are dependent upon an interaction of the host and environment factors. Though several health problems may be related to factors beyond an individual control; yet the clinical outcomes are significantly influenced by "life style." Style generally denotes a distinctive manner of doing or presenting something. Lifestyle includes the way we live our lives interacting with the environment around us. Besides influencing our physical, mental and social health in relation to known causes of ill-health it has been related to several disorders that might afflict a person in his or her lifetime. Changes related to work pressure; dietary habits and social norms have lead to an increase in diseases like diabetes, hypertension, ischaemic heart disease, cancer, psychosomatic and psychiatric disorders to name a few. Since lifestyle is something that can be altered or influenced, it is imperative for us to look at what is a healthy lifestyle and how it can help in prevention of disease or mitigating the effects of a hostile environment or genetic factors. An excellent example of an eminently preventable serious lifestyle disease besides heart disease is cancer of lung, related to tobacco smoking. Tobacco and alcohol consumption along with sedentary lifestyle and unhealthy food habits are responsible for several health problems and are eminently preventable.

Prevention of disease rather than treatment would be the primary goal for leading a meaningful life. In this direction Dr. R. Kumar and Dr. Meenal Kumar have taken a laudable initiative by bringing out a book on "Guide to Total Fitness of Body and Mind." The authors frequently write in the health columns of leading newspapers like the *Tribune* to achieve their objectives of Fitness promotion and Disease prevention. They have already brought out a series of books to promote health, wellness and fitness on a continuing basis. In this book they have not only contributed chapters but have more importantly induced several professionals with impeccable credentials to contribute to this book. It has been written in a simple and lucid style. I believe that this book shall be useful to the lay public as well as the practitioners of medicine. Thus, it will be a great leap forward in supplementing the efforts of clinicians at various levels, including tertiary hospitals like PGI.

I sincerely hope that all of us at individual level would endeavour to have a healthy lifestyle and all practitioners of medicine would make it a mission to promote it. The objective should be positive health through total fitness.

Chandigarh

SUBHASH VARMA
Prof. and Head,
Department of Internal Medicine,
PGIMER, Chandigarh

1

Brain and Nerves: Learn to keep them Healthy and Fit

M. MODI AND S. PRABHAKAR*

INTRODUCTION

With recent improvements in maternal and child healthcare and advances in the treatment of infectious diseases, neurological disorders have emerged as a priority health issue world-wide. Neurological diseases contribute extensively to morbidity and mortality in tropical countries affecting millions every year. Unfortunately effective treatment is available for only a few of these disorders. Moreover, many of these diseases are left with unacceptable sequelae, resulting in severe disability. There are a number of physical and social problems that are faced by these physically handicapped persons, which need to be addressed. It is therefore pertinent that effective measures are taken to prevent these diseases wherever possible. Though detailed discussion on individual disorders is beyond the scope of this

* Professor & Head, Department of Neurology, Postgraduate Institute of Medical Education and Research, Chandigarh.

text, an effort has been made to discuss preventive aspects of some of the following common neurological disorders:

Stroke	Nutritional disorders
Epilepsy	Disorders related to Neurotoxins
Headache	Inherited diseases
Infectious Diseases	Neurorehabilitation

STROKE

Stroke is the second leading cause of death after ischaemic heart disease world-wide, accounting for about 5.5 million deaths annually. From a population perspective several risk factors have been identified that if controlled effectively, can result in major reductions in stroke incidence. (Table 1) High blood pressure is the single most powerful risk factor for stroke. Interventions that reduce population-wide blood pressure levels such as program that result in weight loss or reduced salt intake are therefore likely to have major effects on stroke incidence. For example, it has been estimated that a 2% reduction in average world-wide diastolic blood pressure levels would lead to avoidance of about half a million stroke deaths per year in Asia alone. Other modifiable determinants of initial stroke risk include smoking and diabetes mellitus, which are highly prevalent in developing countries. Management of stroke epidemics in such countries require major efforts to reduce smoking and prevent the weight gain that leads to diabetes and atherosclerosis. Also, dietary modifications may need to be done to control obesity and dyslipidemia.

Secondary Prevention

Patients with identifiable risk factors and family history of atherosclerosis may be considered for prophylactic aspirin. In a meta analysis, use of aspirin was found to be associated with 13% risk reduction for recurrent vascular events. There had been considerable debate regarding appropriate dose of aspirin for prevention of stroke, the recent trials supporting the use of lower doses (75-300 mg/day). Recently ESPS-2 trial has shown that the combination therapy of low dose aspirin

TABLE I

Risk Factors for Ischaemic Stroke

Well Documented	*Less Well Documented*
Modifiable	**Potentially modifiable**
Hypertension	Insulin resistance
Smoking	Obesity
Diabetes	Physical inactivity
Carotid stenosis	Excess alcohol consumption
Transient ischaemic attacks	Hormone replacement therapy
Sickle cell disease	Oral contraceptives
Atrial fibrillation	Lipid abnormalities (i.e. low HDL, high LDL)
Myocardial infarction	Illicit drug use
Congestive heart failure and cardiomyopathy	Hypercoagulability (eg. Factor V Leiden def.)
Valvular disease	Inflammation (measured by C-reactive protein)
	Infectious agents (i.e., C. pneumoniae, H. pylori and cytomegalovirus)
Potentially modifiable	Dietary factors
Diabetes	Migraine
Hyperhomocysteinemia	Socio-economic factors.
Non-modifiable	
Age	
Race/ethnicity	
Gender	
Hereditary/genetic factors	
Geographic location	
Climate and seasonal variations	

Key: HDL—High Density Lipoprotein; LDL—Low Density Lipoprotein.

(50 mg/day) with dipyridamole (400 mg/day) is more beneficial than use of either drug alone. The relative risk reduction of stroke was 37% with combination therapy, 21.2% with aspirin alone and 19.4% by dipyridamole alone, as compared to placebo.

Patients with atrial fibrillation are at increased risk for stroke and have been targeted for both primary and secondary prevention strategies. The presence of additional risk factor like TIA, hypertension, congestive heart failure, diabetes and age more than 75 years, greatly increases stroke risk in these patients. As per ACP guidelines, warfarin therapy is indicated in all high risk patients with AF, regardless of age and for all patients above 75 years of age regardless of the risk. Patients below 65 years of age, without risk factors can be treated with aspirin alone. In those between 65 and 75 years of age, choice depends on physicians' preference and underlying medical conditions.

In a recent review of all trials of cholesterol lowering agents in primary and secondary prevention of stroke, a significant reduction in stroke risk was found in persons treated with statin agents. Recently hyperhomocysteinemia has been proposed as an important risk factor for atherosclerotic vascular disease including stroke. Whether lowering of homocysteine levels reduce the incidence of stroke is still debated, fortification of food with folic acid or oral supplementation of B-vitamins (B1, B6 and B12) are simple and effective measures to reduce homocysteine levels.

EPILEPSY

The prevalence of epilepsy throughout the world varies from 4 to 10 per 1000 population. Established risk factors for epilepsy which are important in developing countries include head injury, infections, infestations and toxins. Mental retardation, cerebral palsy and seizures are important associated conditions. In a recent population-based study from Chandigarh, history of head injury, febrile seizure, developmental delay and a family history of epilepsy ware found to be significant risk factors. Poverty and illiteracy in tropical zones promote malnutrition, poor sanitation and high prevalence of infections. HIV is emerging as a major health problem in the developing countries and is likely to increase the burden of epilepsy both primarily due to HIV and secondarily due to intracranial infections. About 60% of HIV patients have seizures at some point of the illness.

Based on this data it is clear that many of these epilepsies are preventable. Better antenatal care, intrapartum monitoring and neonatal resuscitation can prevent many a children from developing epilepsy. In developing countries, febrile seizures are often prolonged due to delay in access to good medical care, with possible permanent brain damage and consequent future epilepsy. The use of per rectal diazepam for prolonged febrile seizures needs to be stressed rather than diazepam administered orally or intramuscularly. Improvement of sanitary conditions, and prevention of meningoencephalitis in general and particularly is susceptible individuals can also prevent a large number of individuals from developing epilepsy as sequalae. Routine use of helmets while driving by enforcement or by health education can also reduce the incidence of post-traumatic epilepsy.

Moreover psychosocial issues are frequently most troublesome for patients. Major psychological problems like behavioural disturbances, overprotective and fearful attitude of family members and non-supportive attitude of school authorities affect education at the very foundation. Other major social issues concerning epilepsy are treatment, employment, marriage and pregnancy. One of the major deterrents to effective management is improper treatment of seizures. Orthodox beliefs and thoughts make the patients run to quacks and work on evil spirits rather than taking proper medical treatment and effective antiepileptic drugs. There is a need for proper education and awareness of the patients and their relatives about the disease, its myths the various treatment modalities and the need to take appropriate medical therapy. Unemployment is a major concern in patients with epilepsy. Employers usually reject such patients for fear of recurrence of seizures. The problem can be handled by education, understanding and sympathetic attitude on the part of employer.

Another major sphere of concern in epileptic patients is marriage and pregnancy. The parents usually have difficulty in revealing the fact for the fear of not getting a suitable match and if revealed later, there is a likelihood of her being maltreated. So it is advisable that the girls are well educated and made independent financially and socially. The other family should be explained about the nature of the illness and likelihood of a recurrence rather than hiding the fact. During pregnancy, the patient and family members are apprehensive about the effects of drugs on fetus. They should be adequately counseled about the risks and benefits of the drugs, adverse effects of the seizures to the patient and need for compliance. Use of folic acid supplements, education programmes and follow-up with ultrasonography can lead to a good outcome in most patients

HEADACHE

This is one of the commonest neurological ailments affecting the humans world over. Primary headache syndromes constitute the major bulk and commonly occur in the following forms : migraine with and without aura, tension type headaches, chronic daily headache, cluster headaches, etc. These disturbances cause immense physical, mental and social impact on an individual's life and provide an important target for public health interventions. Many potential triggers have been studied in migraine causation, although the cause and effect relationship is not entirely proven. These can be classified into : behavioural (fasting, emotions, sleep problems, stress, exercise); environmental (light, odours, weather changes, cigarette smoke); infections (URI); dietary (caffeine, alcohol, aged cheese, chocolate, ice cream, etc.); chemical (monosodium glutamate, tyramine, nitrates, aspartame); hormonal, etc. These triggers can be minimized by lifestyle modifications, e.g. limiting caffeine consumption, maintaining regular sleep hygiene, eating regularly and avoiding fasting, minimizing stress, exercise and relaxation techniques and avoidance of bright lights. Adequate treatment through a regular medical advise rather than using frequent 'over the counter' medications would prevent analgesic abuse and worsening clinical picture.

Many patients may be helped by behavioural and other non-pharmacological treatments. Behavioural therapy can increase the effectiveness of pharmacotherapy and prevent overuse and misuse of analgesics. Relaxation therapies, biofeedback, acupuncture, nutritional approaches, exercise schedules, aroma therapy, etc are alternative therapies with the aim of reducing frequency and severity of headaches and necessity for drugs. They also carry the potential for prevention of the occurrence of headaches.

INFECTIOUS DISEASES OF NERVOUS SYSTEM

1. Bacterial diseases
2. Parasitic
3. Helminthic
4. Viral

BACTERIAL DISEASES

Common bacterial diseases including pyogenic meningitis, neurotuberculosis, tetanus, neurosyphilis and leprosy will be discussed in the text.

A. Pyogenic Meningitis

Pneumococus, H. influenzae and meningicoccal meningitis are the major causes of pyogenic meningitis world-wide and account for 75 to 80% of all cases. The most important site of entry of these organisms to blood stream and subsequently to the CSF is via the upper respiratory track. Of these, meningococci are the major cause of epidemics of bacterial meningitis world-wide. Household crowding, living in military barracks, poverty and lack of education are some of the factors associated with increased incidence of meningitis.

Preventive measures include avoidance of over-crowding and isolation of known cases of meningitis. Chemoprophylaxis is advisable for household contacts of both N. menigitides and H. influenzae meningitis cases. Rifampicin is presently the drug of choice and should be given to the index case also. More definitive preventive measures include vaccination.

(i) Meningococcal Vaccine

Polysaccharide vaccines are available against meningococci of the A, C, T and W-135 groups. They are recommended for military recruits, patients with terminal complement deficiencies, asplenic patients, alcoholics and people travelling to endemic areas. In epidemics mass vaccination needs to be done.

(ii) Pneumococcal Vaccine

The vaccines are given to adults and children predisposed to pneumococcal infection.

(iii) H. influenzae Vaccine

The vaccine is conjugated with immunogenic protein, resulting in good response evén is infancy and has a considerable impact on the incidence of this infection.

B. Neurotuberculosis

Infection with Mycobacterium tuberculosis is common in developing countries. There are approximately three million infectious cases and 12 million non-infectious cases of tuberculosis in India, resulting in over half a million deaths every year. The incidence of tubercular meningitis varies from 7-12%. Intracranial tuberculomas constituted 20-30% of all intracranial space occupying lesions in previous studies which is now progressively declining. Potts' spine is the commonest cause of cord compression leading to paraplegia in tropics. With the advent of AIDS, there is resurgence of tuberculosis. It is estimated that 50% or more of tuberculosis complicating AIDS is associated with extrapulmonary involvement, brain being the commonest site. Clinical Presentation depends on the underlying pathology like chronic meningitis, tuberculomas or arachnoiditis.

Though the disease cannot be totally prevented, general preventive measures like reduced exposure to active case, good nourishing diet, environmental cleanliness, avoidance of alcohol are general measures to improve body's resistance and prevent tuberculosis. BCG vaccination plays significant role in prevention of tuberculosis, as there is evidence that it does prevent serious and often fatal form of tuberculosis in children, hence the policy of BCG at birth must continue. Chemoprophylaxis with isoniazid for 6-12 months in HIV positive individuals without evidence of active tuberculosis has been tried with promising results.

C. Tetanus

Tetanus almost invariably affects the non-immunised or partially immunised persons or those in whom immunity is waning. More than 1 million patients are affected annually with fatality rate ranging between 20 to 50%. At least half of the deaths occur in neonates, accounting for high mortality in this group. Irony of situation is that the disease is totally preventable. The case of tetanus reflects the failure of health-care delivery system. In developing countries, tetanus continues to be an important health problem due to lack of medical facilities and effective immunisation activities. In addition, illiteracy, unhygienic conditions, unhygienic wound treatment, exposure of wound to soil and hot climates contributes to high incidence. Also inadequate maternal immunization, improper conduct of deliveries, particularly use of contaminated instruments and unhealthy practices especially unclean hands are largely responsible for high incidence of tetanus in rural India.

Tetanus is best prevented by active immunization, as high levels of antibody against tetanus prevent occurrence of tetanus. The aim should be to vaccinate the entire community and ensure a protective level of antitoxin, i.e., 0.01 iu/mg in serum throughout life. It has been seen that the rate of effective levels of antibodies decreases from 57.7% in 6-11 years old to 27.8% in those 70 years or more, hence routine booster immunization is recommended every 10 years. Two preparations are available for active immunization: combined vaccine (DPT) and monovalent vaccine (TT). Tetanus vaccine is offered to all infants under national immunisation programme in combination with diptheria and pertussis vaccine. Three doses of DPT are given at 4-8 weeks' interval, starting at the age of 6 weeks, followed by a first booster dose at 18 months of age, second booster (only DT) at 5-6 years of age and third booster of only TT after 10 years of age. For unimmunized adults three doses are given, first and second 4-8 weeks apart and third dose is given 6 to 12 months after the second dose and a booster is given every 10 years. In unimmunized pregnant women two doses of TT are given in the third trimester, while in previously immunized pregnant women, a booster dose is sufficient.

Prevention strategies following injuries

Injury is the most common mode of acquiring tetanus.

Rarely it may complicate chronic conditions like skin ulcers, eczema, cancerous lesions, gangrene, surgery, middle ear infection, burns or drug abuse. Any breach in skin defences can potentially result in inoculation of tetanus spores. Prophylactic therapy aims at proper management of the wounds, removal of necrotic tissue and foreign body and thorough cleaning of wound. The treatment strategy of wounds is discussed in Table 2 on next page.

For passive immunization human tetanus immunoglobulins (hTIG) is preferable in the dose of 250 to 500 units. When both active and passive immunisations are used simultaneously, separate sites should be chosen using separate syringes. Some patients with humoral immune deficiencies may not respond adequately to toxoid injections. These patients should receive passive immunisation for injuries that carry threat of tetanus.

D. Neurosyphilis

Neurosyphilis was at one time a frequent and disabling disease before the introduction of penicillin therapy. There had been a decline in the prevalence of this disease over the past many decades, till the advent of HIV epidemic. Syphilitic invasion of CNS occurs early in the disease, may be asymptomatically present throughout the entire course of infection and may present as clinical neurosyphilis at any point in the natural history of infection beyond the primary stage. Nearly all cases of syphilis are acquired by sexual contact with infectious lesions (i.e., chancre, mucous patches, skin rash or condyloma latum). Less common modes of transmission include non-sexual personal contact and infection in utero or following blood transfusion.

Hence, the prevention of syphilis depends on the moral values. The awareness of community including sexual education even in school-going children and adolescents will prevent the upcoming epidemic of various STD's. Use of condom should be promoted and public awareness should be brought on these issues. No protective vaccine has been developed till date.

TABLE 2

Treatment Strategy of Wounds

Sl. No.	*Type of wounds*	*Immunization Status*	*Strategy*
1. Clean and minor	Fully immunized Last dose <10 yrs. age	No further treatment	
2. Clean and minor	Unknown immunization history Received fewer than 3 doses of TT	Active immunization Full course of TT	
3. Clean and minor	Received 3 or more doses of TT dose >10 yrs. ago	One dose Tetanus Toxoid	
4. Contaminated and Severe	Fully immunized with last dose <5 yrs. ago	No further treatment	
5. Contaminated and Severe	Fully immunized with last dose >5 yrs. ago	One dose of Tetanus Toxoid	
6. Contaminated and severe	Received 3 or more doses of TT dose >10 yrs. ago	One dose of Tetanus Toxoid, hTIG	
7. Contaminated and severe	Unknown immunisation history Received fewer that 3 doses of TT	Active immunization-TT hTIG	

Secondary Prevention

The early detection and treatment of the disease will go a long way in preventing the ravages of neurosyphilis. Preventive treatment is also recommended for seronegative individuals without signs and symptoms, who have been exposed to infection within the previous three months. Pencillin G. benzathine is the widely used agent for treatment of early syphilis. A single dose of 2-4 million units IM or 1-2 million units in each buttock IM cures more than 95 per cent of cases of primary syphilis. For pencillin allergic patients, a 2 week course of therapy with doxycycline or tetracycline is recommended.

E. Leprosy

Leprosy is a chronic granulomatous infection of human that attack superficial tissues especially the skin and peripheral nerves. This is one of the common causes of peripheral neuropathy world-wide. The site of entry is probably the skin and the mucosa of the upper respiratory track. The chief portal of exit is thought to be nasal mucosa of untreated leprosy patients. Direct human to human transmission is believed to be responsible for most cases of leprosy. Among close family contacts of untreated lepromatous patients, the risk of disease is increased by approximately eight-fold and the attack rate can be as high as 10 per cent. Leprosy remains largely a disease of the rural poor. The number of leprosy cases world-wide has dropped dramatically in the past decade, from an estimated 10 to 12 million cases to 1.8 million cases. Possible contributing factors include improved case detection, use of short course multidrug therapy regimes, BCG vaccination and increasing global urbanization. Case finding and chemotherapy form the basis for the control of leprosy. Early detection of cases is important and requires establishment of local clinics or travelling teams. Family members and other close contacts of cases need to be examined regularly for leprosy. Chemoprophylaxes with dapsone may be effective, but contact screening by yearly physical examination is preferred to empiric therapy. Vaccination with BCG appears to be more effective against prevention of leprosy than that of tuberculosis. Several new vaccines are undergoing field trials, but preliminary results have failed to show significant improvement over BCG.

PARASITIC INFESTATIONS: NEUROCYSTICERCOSIS

Neurocysticercosis (NCC) is the most common parasitic infestation of the CNS world-wide. However, the incidence is highly variable depending on prevailing socio-economic and sanitary conditions. It is still a major public health problem in certain Latin American, African and Asian countries. Cysticercosis is caused by infection with the larval stage of Taenia solium, an intestinal cestode. Certain sites in the body are predisposed to invasion by the parasite, e.g. skeletal muscle, CNS, eye and the subcutaneous tissue. CNS manifestations tend to be highly pleomorphic. Focal or secondary generalized seizures are the commonest presenting features of the disease. Focal deficits, headache and mental changes are seen less frequently. Miliary or the disseminated variety may present with seizures, mental changes and raised intracranial pressure. An encephalitic form mimicking allergic or viral encephalitis may also be seen. A meningitic form resulting in hydrocephalus has been reported more commonly from Mexico. Spinal variety is usually leptomeningeal in type though rarely intramedullary lesions may also be seen. Treatment of Neurocysticercosis requires the use of anti-epileptics, anti-edema measures and in select cases cysticidal drugs like albendazole and praziquantel. Surgical intervention is needed in some patients. Long-term sequelae in the form of epilepsy may result. In some cases dementia and secondary optic atrophy may also ensue.

Cysticercosis is preventable. In order to understand ways in which the lifecycle can be interrupted it is important to know precisely the routes from where this parasite can enter the body system. In the case of T. solium, humans are the only definitive hosts and it inhabits the small intestine. Everyday a few gravid proglottides are detached and excreted in feces. Each of this contains thousands of eggs, which can remain viable for a long time in water and soil. When ingested by the pig these eggs liberate oncospheres, which penetrate the gut wall and enter the blood stream to be subsequently lodged in muscles and other tissues. When humans ingest undercooked pork, these larvae evaginate in the small intestines and grows into adult worms. Cysticercosis results if food contaminated with T. solium eggs is ingested. This also explains incidence of cysticercosis in vegetarians. Adults harboring T. solium can get cysticercosis by either anus to mouth contamination or rarely by autoinfection in which proglottides regurgitate into stomach. Infected food handlers can also transmit infection. Eradication of Taeniasis—cysticercosis cycle should be the ultimate goal and can be achieved by interruption the cycle at various stages. Sanitary inspection of the pork, treatment of waste water before irrigation, and treatment of T. solium carriers are some of the measures, which can help to prevent infection.

PROTOZOAL INFECTION : CEREBRAL MALARIA

Malaria is an endemic problem in tropical countries like India. Cerebral form of disease is being increasingly recognized with emergence of resistance to insecticides and anti-malarials. The clinical manifestations of cerebral malaria are protean and any axis of central nervous system may be implicated in the disease process. Sequelae of the disease can also be disabling and permanent (Table 3). Hence, prompt recognition and correct management are rewarding.

Due to complex life cycle of the parasite the task of designing an effective vaccine has been very difficult. Various types of vaccines against various malarial antigens are being investigated including pre-erythrocytic, merozoite, erythyrocytic and multiple components of malarial parasite. The growing popularity of travel is placing an increasing number of people at risk of malaria. The chemoprophylactic strategies have used various drugs. Chloroquine may be used where its resistance in P. falciparum is not a problem. Mefloquin use has become more widespread due to its favourable anti-malarial activity spectrum and favourable pharmacokinetics that permits once weekly administration. Doxycycline is a worthy alternative agent, though has to be

TABLE 3

Clinical Presentations in Cerebral Malaria

Acute	*Late Sequelae*
Cerebral Disorders	Seizures
Acute febrile encephalopathy	Involuntary movements:
Coma	Dyskinesia/chorea/Parkinsonism
Cranial Nerve Palsies	Multiple sclerosis like presentation
Hemiplegia	Psychiatric syndrome
Paraplegia	Cerebellar syndrome
Spinal disorders	
Myelitis, ALS or Tabes dorsalis like picture	
Peripheral Nerves	
Polyneuritis	
Gulliane-Barre like picture	
Acute Psychiatric manifestations	
Neurasthenia	
Malarial psychosis	

taken once daily. However, no chemoprophylactic can obviate the requirement of effective personal protective measures like use of nets, insect repellants, general environmental cleanliness, regular sprays and other insect controlling manouvres.

VIRAL INFECTIONS OF CNS

A. HIV Infection

First recognised in early 80's in Africa the epidemic of HIV infection continues to spread almost unabated across the world. The infection is associated with a very high morbidity and mortality particularly in the underdeveloped countries where resources and health-care facililties are limited. The main mode of transmission in developing countries is through heterosexual spread, accounting for more than 80% of all cases, while perinatal transmission and blood transfusion contributed about 10% each Homosexual practices and intravenous drug abuse are other less common modes of transmission in developing countries. HIV has been found to be neurotropic, neuroinvasive and neurovirulent and these biological properties play a major role in primary neurological disease. Also the patients become susceptible to a variety of organism including viruses, bacteria, fungi and parasites. The common neurological problems of early and late HIV infection are tabulated (Table 4).

Though large number of antretroiviral agents have been introduced recently and the combination chemotherapy is quite effective, but the cost of therapy is high. Hence, the issue of prevention of HIV infection is so important in tropical countries. The prevention of HIV infection rotates around two strategies. The change of sexual behaviour and development of effective vaccine. The widely advocated use of condoms is not practical in most tropical countries as many of these patients have never seen condom and cannot afford to buy them even when these are provided as cheap as possible. Counselling and health education programmes should deal with this problem effectively. The biology of the virus with its ability to mutate at ease is yet to be fully understood hence the arrival of an effective vaccine is still an unrealistic strategy. The best approach would be change of sexual behaviour among people, promote effective treatment for the STD's and proper screening of blood products before transfusion.

B. Rabies

Inspite of the tremendous advances in therapeutics rabies is still synonymous with death. The epidemiology of rabies varies in different parts of the world and roughly parallels the strict implementation of public health programmes to control domestic rabies. Whereas about one case per year is seen in USA, it still is quite rampant in the third world countries like India, accounting for more than 25,000 cases annually. Dogs are the principle reservoir and the major cause of human rabies. However, bites of other

Table 4

Common Neurological Problems of Early and Chronic HIV Infection

Acute HIV Infection	*Chronic HIV Infection*
Encephalitis	Diffuse brain disease
Delirium	AIDS dementia complex
Acute psychosis	Metabolic/toxic encephalopathies
	Cytomegalovirus encephalitis
Meningitis	Herpes encephalitis
Aseptic meningitis	
Headache/retroorbital pain	Focal brain disease
Recurrences	Toxoplasmosis
	Cryptococcoma
Peripheral neuropathy	Primary CNS lymphoma
Radiculopathy	Secondary deposits
Guillain-Barre syndrome	Progressive multifocal leukoencephalopathy
Transverse myelitis	
	Meningitides
Cranial neuropathies	Aseptic meningitis
Facial palsy	Cryptococcal meningitis
	Syphilitic meningitis
Herpes zoster	Tuberculous meningitis
Cognitive/affective impairment	Spinal cord disease
	Transverse myelitis
	Vacuolar myelopathy
	Herpes myelitis
	Cytomegalovirus myelitis
	Peripheral nerve disease
	Acute/chronic demyelinating polyneuropathy
	Mononeuritis multiplex
	Distal sensory neuropathy
	Herpes zoster neuropathy
	Autonomic neuropathy
	Iatrogenic neuropathy
	Muscle disease
	Inflammatory myopathy (polymyositis)
	Noninflammatory myopathies
	Toxic myopathies

animals like foxes, wolf, jackals, unimmunized domestic cats can also result in rabies. Aerosol transmission and human-to-human transmission by corneal transplants are other uncommon modes of transmission. After a variable incubation period ranging from days to years, the clinical course sets in. Prodromal stage heralds the onset of disease and lasts for 4-10 days. Early features of encephalitis like hyperactivity and bizarre behaviour progresses to the full-blown picture characterized by hydrophobia, autonomic dysfunction, muscle spasms, brainstem dysfunction and coma. Death is inevitable result. A less common form of rabies is the paralytic rabies which resembles Landry Guillaine Barre syndrome. Ante mortem diagnosis is achieved by demonstrating rabies antigen in skin biopsies from neck, corneal impression smear, saliva using fluorescent antibody technique or detection of rabies antibodies either as rising serum or CSF titers. The only effective treatment of rabies is prevention. Extensive health education is required for the general public about the nature of the disease. Control of stray dogs can serve as a ideal deterrent. Unfortunately, the absence of comprehensive national canine rabies control programme in developing countries like India makes control of rabies very difficult. Ignoring post-exposure preventive measures because of wide-spread socio-cultural beliefs and household remedies makes things only worse.

The single most effective measure against rabies virus infection is rigorous cleaning of bite wound in an exposed individual. Use of high concentration of soap or detergent along with antiseptic solution (povidone iodine) is of immense value. Rabies immunoglobulin (RIG) should be administered in high-risk cases after local wound toilet. Human RIG is administered in a dose of 20 IU/kg whereas the less expensive equine RIG is administered in a dose of 40 IU/kg. Half of the doze is infiltrated at the local wound site and half administered intramuscularly. Both vaccine and immunoglobulin must be administered together at separate sites for complete safety. Conventional vaccines are crude preparations of infected brain tissue from sheep, goats or rabbits and can result in serious neurological sequelae. The incidence of neuroparalytic accidents following vaccination varies between 1 in 600 to 1 in 2500. The complications can be major in the form of encephalitis, myelitis, polyradiculitis, meningitis or minor like fever, myalgias and skin reactions. Purified chick embryo vaccine and human diploid cell vaccine (HDCV) are most costly. Reactions to HPCV are uncommon. The administration schedule of HDCV is five one ml doses administered intramuscularly in the deltoid area started as soon as possible and subsequently on 3, 7, 14 and 28 days after initial immunization. Booster dose is administered at the 90th day. Pre-exposure prophylaxis is indicated for individuals with high risks having continuous exposure to rabies virus.

C. Measles

Measles is a highly contagious childhood illness caused by an RNA virus of the paramyxovirus family. Prior to the wide-spread use of vaccination, epidemics used to occur in late winter and early spring months. Malnutrition and lower economic status are important factors, which influence the disease pattern. Unimmunized children are the primary targets of this disease, which is transmitted primarily by aerosolized droplets. Typical clinical features evolve after an incubation period of approximately 10 days. They consist of a prodromal phase, an eruptive phase and a phase of convalescence. Two dreaded neurological complications that can appear are encephalitis during the acute stage and a remote complication known as sub-acute sclerosing panencephalitis (SSPE). Symptoms of encephalitis appear during acute illness, most often during the exanthem. SSPE is caused by an unusual delayed response to persistent infection with measles virus. A defective measles virus maturation in the neural cells results in viral proteins and nucleic acid persisting as defective particles. SSPE usually affects children and adolescents and rarely occurs beyond 18 years of age. There is typically a history of measles infection, often in the first 2 years of life, followed by an asymptomatic period of 6 to 8 years. The illness passes through various stages, which starts with decline in school performance. This is followed by a more pronounced decline in intellectual functions, seizures, myoclonus, ataxia and visual disturbances. In the last stages the child is virtually decorticated and eventually succumbs to the illness. The diagnosis is corroborated by characteristic EEG changes and presence of neutralizing antibodies in the serum and CSF. No effective treatment modality is available. It is prudent therefore that effective preventive measures be taken to limit the occurrence of this unfortunate illness. In the developed countries like U.S.A. with widespread use of vaccine, this illness has practically disappeared. However, in the developing countries like India, the incidence continues to be high. This is presumably the result of high rate of clinical and sub-clinical infections in the young. Measles is best prevented by active immunization. As humans are the only known reservoirs of measles virus, global eradication is possible. The live attenuated vaccine that is currently available is both safe and effective. However, the timing of vaccination is debatable. Too early an administration runs the risk of lack of efficacy due to maternal antibodies while delaying the vaccine can expose these children to risk of acquiring measles. In addition, booster doses may be used to enhance the immunity.

D. Poliomyelitis

Poliomyelitis is characterized by aseptic meningitis and lytic infection of anterior horn cells of the spinal cord leading to transient or permanent paresis of one or more extremities. Improved sanitary conditions and introduction of salk inactivated poliovirus vaccine followed by Sabin oral poliovirus vaccine (OPV) has virtually eliminated poliomyelitis from the developed countries. Poliomyelitis however continues to be endemic in many parts of the world including India. Low level of public concern and poor acceptance of vaccination are some of the major obstacles. Besides this interruption in supply and maintenance of cold chains of the vaccines are other factors. Three poliovirus serotypes have been recognized. Transmission occurs through household contacts and increases with low socio-economic status. More than 90% of the patients have sub-clinical infection.

CNS symptoms consist of aseptic meningitis and asymmetrical motor weakness, the latter being a hallmark of poliomyelitis. As no treatment is available, prevention is the key. Two types of vaccines are available, live attenuated poliovirus vaccine and the inactivated poliovirus vaccine. Both have their merits and demerits. OPV is more suitable for the developing countries like India because of its lower cost, ease of administration, superior local immunity in the gastrointestinal tract and transmission of OPV from immunized to non-immune contacts. In spite of the expanded programme of immunization there are still many stumbling blocks which prevent full protection. Concurrent diarrheal illnesses, malnutrition, vaccine formulation and improper maintenance of cold chains are some of them. Another strategy that has been adopted successfully is the pulse immunization as a supplementation to national immunization schedule. In some countries it has been credited with the abatement of naturally occurring poliovirus and disappearance of disease.

E. Tropical Spastic Paraplegia

Tropical spastic paraplegia or HTLV-1 associated myelopathy is found in many parts of the world with main foci being in the Caribbean, Seychelles islands, South-west of Japan, some parts of Africa and South America. Cases have also been reported from India. HTLV-1 is a retrovirus that is also associated with adult T-cell malignancies. The main routes of transmission are breast feeding, sexual transmission and through blood transfusion. A chronic myelitis causing spastic paraparesis and variable sensory and sphincteric disturbances develops. It has an insidious onset and a slowly progressive course. The CSF may show mild pleocytosis. Blood examination shows elevation of ESR and presence of lobulated lymphocytes. MRI may show atrophy of the cord and hyper intense signal on T2W images. In addition, serological tests in the blood and CSF may be helpful in confirming the diagnosis. In the absence of any effective treatment prevention should be the most important goal. Avoiding promiscuous contacts, use of condoms, screening of blood, and avoidance of breast-feeding in case of infected mothers are some of the preventive measures, which can help in limiting the spread of this disease.

F. Japanese Encephalitis (JE)

JE results from infection of the CNS by an RNA flavivirus. It has been recognized as a distinct disease entity ever since the large epidemic that occurred in Japan in 1924. Presently, cases of JE are known to occur throughout most of Asia. It occurs both as epidemics and as sporadic cases. JE virus is transmitted by culex mosquitoes. The most important reservoirs are pigs and wandering birds and ducks. The life cycle is maintained by transmission between the susceptible vertebrate and the blood-sucking mosquitoes. The disease predominates in the agricultural rural areas. The estimated world-wide incidence of JE is 35,000 to 45,000 cases per year. The disease has an incubation period of 6-16 days. The disease then successively passes through a prodromal phase, an encephalitis phase, phase of defervescence and a convalescent stage. Unfortunately 25% of the affected individuals die and 50% develop sequelae

Treatment of the disease is primarily symptomatic. It is therefore crucial to adopt aggressive prevention measures. An inactivated JE vaccine is available. It should be given to resident population in endemic areas and to travellers at risk. For primary immunization two doses of vaccine are given subcutaneously 1 to 4 weeks apart to children 1-3 yrs. of age. A booster is given after 1 yr. and 3 yrs. Other preventive measures include control of mosquito vector by use of insecticides, mosquito nets and repellants. Vaccination of pigs and other mammals and monitoring JE infections in reservoir animals are other ways to help break the links in transmission. However, such large scale measures are practically impossible in developing countries at present.

G. Creutzfeldt-Jakob Disease (CJD)

CJD is a slow virus infection caused by unconventinal infectious pathogens known as prions. The disease is known to occur world-wide with a prevalence of 0.5-0.8 cases per million. This disease occurs as a sporadic, familial or an iatrogenic form. The disease spectrum consists of sub-acute progressive dementia, myoclonus and typical EEG changes. There is no effective treatment available and the disease invariably has a fatal outcome within 1 year of its onset.

Inherited subset of the disease can be prevented if the affected families undergo prenatal DNA screening and genetic counseling. Iatrogenic transmission has occurred in some cases after transplantation or cornea and dural grafts from infected persons and after implantation of infected depth electrodes. Injection of human growth hormone or gonadotropins prepared from autopsies has also resulted in CJD. In order to reduce the occurrence of this deadly disease safety measures need to be taken. Although barrier nursing is not required, gloves should be worn while handling body fluids. Needles and glassware should be handled carefully and appropriately disinfected and autoclaved or incinerated.

NUTRITIONAL DISORDERS

Nutritional deficiency is still a serious world-wide problem despite great advances since the turn of the twentieth century. Kwashiorkor and marasmus are endemic in most of the underdeveloped countries, while the problem in western countries is usually the result of dietary insufficiency from chronic alcoholism or malabsorption states from gastrointestinal (GI) disorders. Of more than 40 nutrients recognised till date, vitamins are the most significant to neurologists. Although deficiency of almost any vitamins has been reported to produce neurological symptoms, of some kind, the B vitamins, vitamin E and folic acid are the most important. Most causes of nutritional deficiency, whether dietary or malabsorptive do not selectively deplete a single vitamin and results in overlapping neurological syndromes. Undernutrition causes a wide spectrum of neurological disorders, ranging from isolated optic neuropathy to diffuse damage of peripheral and central nervous system (Tables 5 and 6). One of the commonest nutritional disorder is protein energy malnutrition (PEM) which affects upto 3.8% of preschool children in India. Neuropsychological affection is one of the hallmarks of CNS involvement. Cognitional and abstractional abilities are one of the most severely affected. Additional involvement of peripheral nervous system can result in delay in attaining motor milestones in association with severe PEM. The earlier the treatment started, the better is the recovery. The prevention of these disorder lies in provision of adequate and nutritious food to the poor, especially children. This requires a lot of social and political commitment. Peripheral neuropathy is the another common nutritional neurological disorder, that can occur with deficiency of many vitamins.

TABLE 5

Nutritional Deficiencies Associated Neurological Disorders

Sl.. No.	Deficient nutrients	Neurological syndromes
1.	Protein and calories	Kwashiorkor and marasmus
2.	Thiamine	Beriberi, wernicke-korsakoff syndrome
3.	Nictotinic acid	Pellagra
4.	Pyridoxine	Encephalopathy, seizure, neuropathy
5.	Folate	Myelopathy, neuropathy, dementia
6.	Iodine	Cretinism
7.	Vitamin D	Myopathy

In addition to malnutrition, ignorance, dietary faddism, alcoholism, malabsorption, increased requirements like pregnancy are some of the causes of these deficiency states. Hence, timely intervention in the form of education, vitamin supplementation during pregnancy and campaign against alcoholism and other addictions with the help of NGO's and health officials can go a long way is preventing these easily preventable disorders.

DISORDERS OF NERVOUS SYSTEM RELATED TO TOXIN EXPOSURE

Neurotoxic disorders are occurring increasingly as a result of occupational or environmental exposure to chemical agents and often go unrecognised. Known neurotoxins produce stereotyped neurological disturbances that generally cease to progress after exposure is discontinued. Dysfunction of any part of the central, peripheral or autonomic nervous system and of the neuromuscular apparatus may result from

TABLE 6

Neurological Manifestations in Deficiency Diseases

Sl. No.	*Neurological Manifestations*	*Nutritional Deficiencies*
1.	Dementia	Vitamin B12, Nicotinic acid, thiamine, folate
2.	Seizures	Pyridoxine
3.	Myelopathy	Vitamin B12, Vitamin E, folate
4.	Myopathy	Vitamin D, Vitamin E
5.	Peripheral Neuropathy	Thiamine, Vitamin B12, folate, pyridoxine, Vit. E
6.	Optic Neuropathy	Thiamine, Vitamin B12, folate, pyridoxine, Vit. E

exposure to neurotoxins. Usually neurotoxins cause diffuse rather than focal or lateralised neurological dysfunction. Table 7 enumerates the important neurological syndromes caused by exposure to various neurotoxins.

A. Organophosphorus Compounds

Organophosphorus compounds are commonly used insecticides. Exposure may occur while spraying or while handling via the skin if appropriate protective measures are not taken. Pathogenesis is related to inhibition of the enzyme, Neuropathy Target Esterase (NTE). Cholinergic manifestations dominate the clinical picture in the acute stage. Neurological manifestations in the acute stage range from muscle twitchings, muscle weakness, giddiness, confusion, and depression of respiratory center to coma. Intermediate syndrome can develop 24 to 90 hours after poisoning. It is characterized by weakness of proximal muscles as well as muscles supplied by cranial nerves. A small group of these compounds can cause neuropathy. Polyneuropathy manifests following a latent period of a few weeks. The main features are paresthesias, distal weakness and wasting. Recovery, which is variable, may take up to two years. Workers exposed to pesticides suffer from both acute and low level chronic poisoning. Health education of these ignorant farmers along with the demonstration of proper techniques of handling these pesticides needs to be emphasized.

TABLE 7

Neurotoxins: Site of Damage and Clinical Features

Site of Damage	Clinical Features	Neurotoxic substances
1. Foetal CNS malformation	Anencephaly	Spoiled potato (Glykoalkaloid solanine)
2. Corticospinal tract	Spastic paraplegia	Lathyrus sativus, cassava
3. Myoneural	Muscle weakness	Krait venom, tropical fish toxin curare
4. Basal ganglia	Parkinsonian syndrome	Manganese
5. Spinal cord syndrome	Paraplegia, spastic quadriplegia	Lathyrism, fluorosis
6. Retinal damage: visual loss	Diminished visual activity	Organophosphate, fenthion, triethyline
7. Cortical hyperexcitability	Epileptic fits	Organochlorine pesticide, BHC isomer
8. Auditory cochlear hair cells	Deafness	Cadmium compounds
9. Intracranial cytotoxic oedema	Encephalopathy	Pesticides, lead (in children)
10 Raised ICT	Headache	Solvents, pesticides, lead
11 Limbic system	Behaviour problems, psychosis	Managanese, OPC, cannabis, datura
12 Peripheral nerve	Motor sensory neuropathy	TOCP, lead, arsenic

BHC: Benzahexachlorine, OPC: Organophosphate compounds, TOCP: Triorthocresyl phosphate.

B. Fluorosis

In humans fluoride maintains normal mineralization of bones and prevents teeth from caries. However, in areas where the fluoride content of the water and foodstuffs is high, ingestion of these over prolonged periods leads to a debilitating chronic illness called Fluorosis. The disease occurs with varying intensity in various parts of India like Andhra Pradesh, Tamil Nadu, Mysore, Punjab, etc. The brunt of the disease is borne by the skeletal system. The various factors, which govern the development of Fluorosis, are the total amount of fluoride ingested which depend on the level of fluoride in the food and water, duration of ingestion, nature of work and the nutritional status. Excess of fluoride causes increase in bony mass. Ligaments and muscle attachments also get calcified. The spine ultimately becomes rigid and inflexible. The osteophytes projecting into the spinal canal and intervertebral foramina may press the cord and spinal roots producing the syndrome of myeloradiculopathy at a single or multiple levels. The diagnosis in persons living in endemic areas is not difficult. X-rays of the bones showing increased osteosclerosis, calcification of the ligaments and interosseous membranes and increased fluoride excretion in a 24 hours urinary sample support the diagnosis of Fluorosis. The treatment of Fluorosis is not without difficulties. Prevention is thus the best form of therapy and should be the aim in all cases. Water purifying plants should be installed in endemic areas to reduce the amount of fluoride, which should be kept below 1 ppm in drinking water. Appropriate measures also need to be taken in industries, supplemented with periodic check ups.

C. Lathyrism

Lathyrism is a neurotoxic disorder caused by consumption of Lathyrus sativus. L. sativus is a very piosonous legume, which becomes a survival food for the poor in areas hit by famine and other natural calamities. The disease is seen in certain tropical countries including India, Bangladesh, Ethiopia and China. Prolonged consumption of L. sativus (30% of daily diet over 4 weeks) is usually responsible for the disease. B-N-oxalylamine-L-alanine (BOAA), the responsible free toxic amino acid produces its ill-effects as a result of excitotoxicity. Lathyrism is clinically characterized by a rather pure spastic paraparesis in the absence of other neurological signs. It has been classified as no stick stage, one or two sticks stage and the crawler stage The disease can commence acutely or more slowly. Variable symptoms in the form of paresthesias, urgency and sphincteric spasm may be associated. Lathyrus sativus has actually good nutritional quality except for the presence of BOAA. Development of a non-toxic strain has invoked great interest. Use of non-toxic strains shall enable the poor people in the affected areas to continue its intake. However, till the time this can be done other measures in the form of health education, banning of the crop and measures, which reduce the toxic content need to be taken.

D. Lead

Clinical manifestations of lead toxicity, also known as plumbism, are not uncommon. The common sources of exposure include paints, plumbing, leaded gasoline, batteries and improperly glazed ceramics. Clinical symptomatology is more severe in the childhood. Children can develop irritability and lethargy, which may progress to frank encephalopathy. Deficits in intellectual functions can also appear. In adults peripheral motor neuropathy is a common symptom. Lead toxicity can also have non-neurological manifestations such as anemia, abdominal pain and renal failure. Chelating agents are useful for the treatment though the key lies in the prevention. Occupational safety measures along with regular monitoring of serum lead levels can go a long way in prevention of plumbism.

E. Arsenic

Arsenic is used in many *desi* medications in toxic doses. In Northern India, opium addicts have been found to develop arsenic neuropathy. It is also a contaminant of some deep-water wells. Persons who are on a very high fish based diet may also develop this toxicity. Following acute toxicity there are usually gastrointestinal symptoms. This is followed by neuropathy after a few weeks. Low-level exposure can also result in a predominantly painful sensory axonal neuropathy. Other hallmarks of the disease are the characteristic skin lesions. Mee's lines (transverse gray lines) in the nails, can also be seen. Therapy with chelating agents can benefit but residual deficit may be left. Measures should be taken to limit the exposure to arsenic. In addition, individuals at increased risk of arsenic toxicity should have regular urine check for the level of arsenic.

E. Manganese

Manganese is widely distributed natural resource with India being the third largest producer of manganese. Manganese oxide is used in paint, varnish, fireworks, ink and certain pesticides and fertilizers. Health hazards may arise during mining as an occupational exposure. Manganese toxicity can produce many neuropsychiatric manifestations. A spastic rigid syndrome that mimics parkinsonism is known to develop. Adequate measures need to be taken to prevent its toxicity, particularly in the mine workers.

G. Mercury

Inorganic elemental mercury toxicity results from inhalation during industrial exposure as in battery factories, mercury processing plants, and electronic appliance factories. In past exposure used to occur in hat making industries. Clinically features include erythema, hyperhidrosis, intention tremors (hatter's shake) and personality changes (Mad as a hatter). The organic mercury (methyl and ethyl mercury) are potent neurotoxins causing degnerations in cerebellar granular layer, calcarine cortex, and dorsal root ganglion neurons. Chronic methyl mercury poisoning results in sensory disturbance, constriction of visual fields, progressive ataxia, tremors and cognitive impairment. Few cases resemble ALS. The effects of organic mercury poisoning have come to be widely recognised since outbreak in Minamata Bay (1950) in Japan when industrial waste discharged into the bay led to contamination of fish that were consumed by humans. Presently, it is being used as fungicides in agriculture and in paper industry. Outbreak occur when seeds treated with methyl mercury intended for plantation are consumed. So appropriate measure like use of masks and prevention of exposure of fungicide, in addition to education of the agriculturists are essential in preventing outbreaks.

G. Carbon Monoxide Poisoning

Carbon monoxide is produced in large amounts by incomplete combustion of wood, gasoline engines, tobacco products and in certain industrial processes. It is rapidly absorbed from the lungs and binds to hemoglobin with a higher affinity resulting in tissue hypoxia. Dyspnea, nausea, vomiting, diarrhea, and a host of neuropsychiatric symptoms characterize the acute syndrome. In the advanced stages there may be coma, arrhythmias, hypotension, respiratory depression and pulmonary edema. Oxygen therapy is the mainstay of therapy. The main concern however is the persistence of sequelae in some patients. Bilateral necrosis of the globus pallidus is the pathological hallmark of this disease entity although can be seen in other hypoxic ischemic states as well. The sequelae may consist of gross neurological deficit in the form of parkinsonism, in-coordination, etc. The key to avoiding these complications is prevention. Adequate precautions need to be taken at work places and at homes to avoid these accidents.

INHERITED DISORDERS

There are vast number of neurological diseases with a genetic basis. The various modes of inheritance include single gene (Mendelian), chromosomal, multifactorial and mitochondrial. In addition, many neurological diseases are the result of a combination between a genetic predisposition and an environmental insult. Examples of various inherited disorders include neurofibromatosis, tuberous sclerosis, Huntington's disease, several hereditary ataxias and neuropathies, myotonic dystrophy (all autosomal dominant), Wilson's disease, Fredriech's ataxia (autosomal recessive), Duchenne's and Becker's muscular dystrophies, (X-linked recessive) and Leber's hereditary optic neuropathy (mitochondrial disorders).

Although most of these disorders evoke a lot of clinical curiosity, nothing much can be offered to most of these cases. It is therefore important that preventive measures be taken. In general preventive approach includes genetic screening, counseling and prenatal diagnosis. The screening tests allow for early detection of these cases and provide an opportunity to initiate therapy so that the damage can be minimized.

Genetic counseling deals with problems related to risk of occurence of a genetic disorder in the family. This includes a detailed family history, educating patients, needs, risks, benefits and limitations of genetic testing and medical as well as psychosocial support of the family. It is also indicated in advanced maternal and paternal age, consanguinity, previous history of birth defects or genetic disorder, higher risk ethnic groups, known carriers and ultrasound and prenatal testing suggesting a genetic disorder. Genetic testing aims at either diagnosing, predicting, carrier testing or prenatal testing for the given disorder under consideration. Techniques for antenatal testing include maternal serum analysis (alphafetoprotein, etc.), amniocentesis, chorionic villus biopsy, ultrasonography, and pre-implantation molecular diagnostic testing. It is important to remember that prenatal diagnosis focus on chromosomal abnormalities and specific genetic disorders with high risk of transmission. It is important that parents are explained about limitations and need for the tests. With the immense growth in our understanding of diseases and advent of molecular techniques the physician's task is increasing. The physician must integrate medical history, family history and diagnostic techniques for overall care of these patients.

NEURO REHABILITATION

Significant physical and mental disabilities lead to impairment of occupational and social performance. In India, it is estimated that 3 to 4% of its population is disabled due to one or more health problems. This will amount to 30 to 40 million people requiring rehabilitation. Neurological diseases are responsible for 40 to 50% of their disabilities. In a study conducted by Prabhakar *et al*, it was shown that after 1 year of discharge from hospital, only 40% improved significantly while 29% showed no improvement and 5% had actually worsened. These disabilities may be motor, communicative, visual, hearing or cognitive skills. In addition, these disabilities could be either static, improving or progressive. Keeping in view the large burden of these patients and our limited resources it is imperative that proper allocation of resources and community-based rehabilitation services be done.

As stroke is one of the leading causes of disability, great attention needs to be paid to the often forgotten aspect of rehabilitation. In general, formal rehabilitation measures can be initiated if there has been no progression of neurological illness for 48 hours. The primary goals of early intervention are to prevent intellectual and physical deterioration that may delay subsequent rehabilitation efforts. The basic principles of physical therapy involve preventing or correcting deformity, increasing sensory input to increase motor output, strengthening muscles and applying basic learning concepts so that the patients can rehearse activities. Applying active assisted range of movements (ROM) to sound side and passive ROM to the affected extremities are commenced for better conditioning of the patient. The paralyzed upper extremity is at risk of developing shoulder hand syndrome, glenohumeral subluxation and brachial plexus traction injuries. Care should be taken to prevent these. Subsequent to the acute stage, rehabilitative measures include developing the ability to perform the skills and tasks of daily life. Learning occurs through various stages. The first stage is characterized by frequent errors and variable performance to a final phase when the performance is smoother and automatic. EMG feedback can also be used for up training or down training agonist and antagonist muscles for a specific activity. Treatment of speech and language and cognitive disorders should also be undertaken simultaneously. Post-stroke depression is another major issue, which needs adequate care.

Patients with neuromuscular disorders, present a different subset of problems and challenges. In children with these disorders principles of rehabilitation include optimal physical, mental and emotional improvement, maintaining function as long as possible and preventing secondary complications like contractures. Patients with Duchenne's muscular dystrophy, a common muscular dystrophy, face a number of problems as the disease advances. In addition to weakness contractures cause major problems. Early stretching exercises to prevent contractures of hip flexors, iliotibial bands and heel cord form a very important part of management. Sub-maximal exercises can also be helpful. In addition, muscle-toning exercises are often useful in improving ventilatory endurance, as respiratory failure is a common mode of exit in these patients. The use of braces and surgery to release contractures and correct deformities may be required in the terminal stages. One of the most difficult things faced by physicians is to communicate to the patient and his family about the progressive nature of the diseases and lack of any treatment. It requires lot of communicative skills. The family should be informed about the true nature of the disease without causing significant emotional distress. Patients with the diagnosis of Motor neuron disease (MND) are confronted with a number of problems as the disease progresses. Feeding is particularly a problem and may lead to aspiration. MND patients and their attendants should be informed about the disease with inherent variability of the clinical course along with the knowledge about various palliative therapies that are available to improve the quality of life. Ryle's tube insertion or a percutaneous endoscopic gastrostomy may have to be resorted to. Communication aids may be required to manage dysarthria. Assisted ventilation may be considered for a select group of patients. Patients with hereditary neuropathies need to be given vocational guidance. The most commonly required orthosis to prevent foot drop and contractures. Once the diagnosis of a particular neurological disorder is made and the patient and family have been informed about the true nature of disease, the process of rehabilitation should commence. It should be a multidisciplinary approach comprising of a neurologist, social worker, orthopedic surgeon, physiotherapist, occupational therapist and a geneticist.

2

Maintain Fitness: Prevent Diabetes and other Top Killers

1. INTRODUCTION

Diabetes is a serious disease that can develop from the lack of insulin production in the body or due to the inability of the body's insulin to perform its normal everyday functions. Insulin is a substance produced from the pancreas gland that helps process the food we eat and turn it into energy. Diabetes is usually induced by an unhealthy lifestyle, stress, and is a very treacherous disease. Genes also play a role in its occurrence. It causes no pain but it deteriorates your body over time. That is why most of us don't even know that we have diabetes. If untreated and unmanaged you will die slowly and prematurely. You will start to get circulatory problems, which progress into limb numbness. After that you will get kidney problems resulting in dialysis; and after that retina problems, resulting in blindness. After that your body will disintegrate more and more until you die. . . . It is a horrible and devastating process .The good news is that it doesn't have to be that way. You can live a long, healthy life, savor all the foods you ever dreamt of, go anywhere, and do anything you're capable of—despite diabetes. Eating sensibly, living a healthy lifestyle, getting emotional support, and pursuing your personal dreams are crucial to minimizing complications, and managing diabetes as effectively and efficiently as possible. Diabetes may be a chronic disease, but it only cause "disease" if your blood glucose rises above or falls below the normal range. And keeping your glucose within the normal range is basically up to you. Sure. Your physician, and your family and friends can help. Adopting a healthy diet and attitude of fitness is all about making permanent personal changes. Changes are tough, no doubt about it. But you can be successful—if you make your changes slowly and consciously, one small step at a time. Forget crash diets.

Diabetes disrupts the vascular system, affecting many areas of the body such as the nerves, heart, eyes, kidneys, legs, and feet. People with diabetes need to pay special attention to their feet. The family physician can help a diabetic a lot, since he has frequent contacts with their patients, knows their family history, can encounter pre-symptomatic stage of disease, can influence lifestyle of their patients. The changed lifestyle and an attitude of fitness helps to ward-off not only diabetes, but other top killers as well.

2. SIZE OF THE PROBLEM

Diabetes in Indians has become a problem of great magnitude. It is estimated that between 10-12% of the urban population and 4-6% of the rural population of India now have diabetes. Unfortunately, 25% of urban population is threatened with diabetes, due to rich and excessive food intake, with hardly any exercise. Listed below are the estimated number of diabetics in top 3 countries with diabetes in the world according to recent WHO estimates. It

Nation	*Estimated number of people with diabetes (in millions)*	
	In 1995	*In 2025*
India	19.4	57.2
China	16.0	37.6
U.S.A.	13.9	21.9

can be seen that the number of diabetic patients in India already far exceeds that in China and U.S.

What is more disheartening is that many of the diabetes related complications (e.g., Ischaemic Heart Disease) are also more common among Indians. Furthermore, both diabetes and ischaemic heart disease occur at a younger age (at least a decade earlier) in Indians compared to Europeans. Diabetic retinopathy leading to blindness, Diabetic nephropathy leading to kidney failure and Diabetic foot disease leading to amputations also take a heavy toll in terms of morbidity of the patient. Luckily a lot can quite easily be done to prevent the morbidity and mortality associated with diabetes. Of paramount importance is early detection and diagnosis of the disease. One should remember that diabetes is a very silent disease and is often asymptomatic. Hence, regular screening for diabetes is the only way to detect diabetes at an early stage.

Given the very high prevalence of diabetes in our country, it would be advisable for everyone above the age of 30 years (and above 20 years in those with a strong family history of diabetes) to have the first check-up for diabetes, which should ideally be a Glucose Tolerance Test (GTT). If diabetes is detected at early stages, e.g. at the stage of Impaired Glucose Tolerance, it may be possible to halt the progression to overt diabetes or indeed, even reverse the natural history to a normal glucose tolerance stage. Even in those with no evidence of diabetes it is better to repeat the test at least once a year.

Family history	*Risk of Diabetes*
If both parents are diabetic	99%
One parent diabetic and any other relative of non-diabetic parent is also diabetic	75%
If one parent is diabetic	50%
Any other close relative	25%

After diabetes has set in, one should strive to achieve good control of diabetes continuously. Unfortunately, being a life long disorder, many patients tend to neglect it after an initial period of good control.

Test	*Period of diabetic control assessed*
Blood sugar	Instantaneous
Urine sugar	Previous 3-4 hours
24 hours urine sugar	Previous 24 hours
Fructosamine	Previous 2-3 weeks
Glycosylated hemoglobin	Previous 2-3 months
Retinal (eye) examination	Previous 5-10 years (approx.)

Methods used to Assess Diabetic Control

At home, the patient can test his urine sugar using Benedict's Solution or one of the strip tests. Today, it is also possible for the patient to test his blood sugar accurately using small meters which are getting smaller, less expensive and more patient-friendly, every day. In addition, the patient also needs to periodically visit their doctor or a diabetes specialist. An annual check-up of the eyes, kidneys, heart and feet is mandatory in order to detect complications (if present) at an early stage. Additional tests of the nerves and other organs can also be done whenever necessary. Keeping a tab on the serum cholesterol including its various sub-fractions like LDL and VLDL (bad cholesterol), HDL (good cholesterol) and triglycerides is also essential. Regular check-up of the blood pressure and body weight will also help to keep complications at bay. The two main pillars in the management of diabetes still remain diet and exercise. Improvements in diabetic medications both tablets and insulin and improved methods of insulin delivery systems have also made control of diabetes much easier today than in yesteryears. Needless to say, the patient also has to do his part and this includes strict diet and regular exercise. All these methods when judiciously combined together will make the diabetic's life a fuller and healthier one. Low levels of activity, resulting in fewer calories used than consumed, contribute to the high prevalence of obesity in the United

States.

- Physical activity may favourably affect body fat distribution. People of all ages, both male and female, benefit from regular physical activity.
- More than 60 percent of American adults are not regularly physically active. In fact, 25 percent of all adults are not active at all.
- Significant health benefits can be obtained by including a moderate amount of physical activity on most, if not all, days of the week.
- Additional health benefits can be gained through greater amounts of physical activity.
- Physical activity reduces the risk of premature mortality in general, and of coronary heart disease, hypertension, colon cancer, and diabetes mellitus in particular.

Physical activity also improves mental health and is important for muscles, bones and joints.

India has highest number of diabetics and most of them remain undetected and untreated due to ignorance and poverty, thus leading to many complications and resultant high incidence of death and disability. We are heading towards an epidemic of this non-communicable disease. Diabetes with vascular complications is the most frequent cause of death of middle-aged patients and the leading cause of the long-term morbidity and disability. The prevalence of coronary heart disease, lower limb ischemia and stroke is 5-6 times higher compared with the non-diabetic population. Higher attention must therefore be given to people at the highest risk to develop such disease. The most frequent causes of death and disability of the diabetic patients are:

A. Heart attacks due to ischemic heart disease
B. Infections
C. Stroke
D. Foot gangrene
E. Renal insufficiency
F. Blindness due to retinopathy

Primary health care needs to focus its screening activity on people with increased risk of diabetes mellitus. This means particular attention to the subjects above 40 years of age with familial predisposition to diabetes mellitus and a family history of hypertension, heart disease, stroke, ischemic disease of the lower limbs. Moreover, patients suffering from hypertension, dyslipidaemia, obesity, gout or hyperuricaemia and gestation diabetes are special targets for preventive approach. To realise early detection, continuous education of patients and their families is required. In addition, their offspring need BMI assessment measurement; Casual glycaemia once a year; Checking for albuminuria; Examination of serum lipids; Checking blood pressure, assessment for Obesity (BMI > 27), assessment for Manifest heart and vascular disease. If abnormal results are found a more intense follow-up programme is needed.

3. ASIAN EXPERIENCES

In India many studies have been carried out, which have led us to conclude that the incidence of diabetes is rising fast due to lethargic lifestyle, unimaginative over-eating and lack of attitude for fitness. Manifestation of complications is however influenced by one's lifestyle and food intake. Punjab is a living example, where more and more people are taking to western style of fat rich food and relatively sedentary style of life, many of them have developed heart disease and diabetes at a younger age. In a Malaysian study food intake both in terms of quantity and the type of foods have been identified as the major influencing factor in the development and management of diabetes. A healthy lifestyle is generally taken to mean having a closely knitted family life, having hobbies that are healthy physically and mentally, away from drug abuse and the kicking of the habit of excessive drinking or smoking. Excessive food intake is seldom feature. In recent years, it is recognised that excessive food intake invariably leads to many health problems and diabetes is one such example. In Malaysia, statistically, in 1986 some 6.8% of the population were diabetics. Today, the figure has increased to 8% and is believed to be growing. The figure could actually be higher than this as there are many who may be suffering from the problem but go undetected. In fact, there are similar trend in the newly developed nations of South East Asia such as Singapore and Hong Kong. The cause of this rising incidence of diabetes is attributed by most authorities to the increasing affluence of the society, the changing of lifestyle, the higher consumption of fine foods and down right over consumption of foods—a price that we pay for the booming economy. Early detection of the condition is the best way of preventing development of complications. As the saying goes, prevention is better than cure, although it is not possible to prevent the development of diabetes altogether, with the correct dietary habit and exercise its onset may be delayed. The suffering as a result of complications arising from neglect can largely be avoided and a patient can expect to live a near normal and good qualify life.

Obesity has become more prevalent; food energy availability has generally risen beyond requirements with a trend towards increased sugar consumption. Life expectancy has been progressively increasing over the last thirty years in the Region, reaching in some countries figures, which are similar to those seen in the industrialized world.

In a study in Pakistan, it was concluded that physical inactivity, obesity and fat distribution over the abdomen have emerged as the major causes of deterioration of glucose tolerance. Thus, primary prevention of diabetes can be achieved by decreasing insulin resistance through correction of obesity and increased physical activity and by the promotion of healthy nutritional trends (reduction in the consumption of fat and refined carbohydrates and increase in fiber content of the diet). The major goal of diabetes management should be to achieve good control of diabetes.

The recent prevalence survey on diabetes mellitus conducted by Diabetic Association of Pakistan in collaboration with WHO shows that diabetes prevalence is over 10% in both sexes in the people aged 25 years or above. Central obesity and positive family history are strongly associated with diabetes. The association of central obesity are greater for women than for men.

4. TYPES OF DIABETES

Type 1: Diabetes or Juvenile Diabetes

This is the typically genetic induced form of diabetes and in most cases stems from an inability of the pancreatic system to produce enough insulin. It usually has to be treated and managed by injecting insulin into your bloodstream. It is the most severe type of diabetes and can be rarely reversed, although there are hopeful signs of research experiments with transplants of pancreatic cells. Fountain of Health can slow the progression and prolong life.

Type 2: Diabetes

This is the most common form of diabetes. It is usually lifestyle induced through overeating, sedentary lifestyle, smoking, junk food, lack of exercise and stress. This lifestyle creates a cell resistance to insulin, leading to high blood sugar levels. It is usually contained and managed by taking oral medication of various strengths. Fountain of Health and especially weight isometrics seems to reduce the cell receptive resistance and allows managing this condition with lower oral medication.

Diabetes Mellitus

This is a chronic form of diabetes involving an insulin deficiency and characterized by excess sugar in the blood and urine, hunger, thirst, and gradual loss of weight.

Insipidus Diabetes

This is usually caused by a pituitary deficiency and characterized by the heavy discharge of urine and intense thirst.

Gestational Diabetes

This is usually caused by pregnancy. It may or may not disappear after pregnancy. It is a red flag and signals a precondition for diabetes development. The Fountain of Health system could be used as a preventative measure.

5. HOW A DIABETIC PATIENT MAY PRESENT

It should be noted that patients with diabetes mellitus might be encountered with the following situations:

- ❑ Urinary infections, often repeated,
- ❑ Pruritis vulvae,
- ❑ Hypertension,
- ❑ Joint diseases associated with obesity,
- ❑ Skin diseases and infections,
- ❑ Mono-neuropathy, neurogenic pain and sensory disorder,
- ❑ Symptoms of CHD, TIA, diseases of lower limbs or stroke, and
- ❑ On steroid treatment.

Physicians need to investigate all the patients with above symptoms as potential diabetic patients. General Practitioners and their co-workers must be aware that cardiovascular complications may already be implicated at the stage of impaired glucose tolerance. To improve the quality of life of persons with diabetes mellitus the following measures are necessary:

1. To promote actively good metabolic control for blood glucose;
2. To promote regular blood pressure control and treatment and lipids;
3. To ensure regular body weight control—BMI;
4. To treat actively urinary infection;
5. To promote healthy lifestyle, e.g. smoking, salt intake, nutrition and exercise;
6. To promote self-care;
7. To promote shared care with regular assessment and therapeutic intervention by an ophthalmologist, neurologist and cardiologist;
8. To refer to the diabetologist in case of insufficient metabolic compensation of diabetes mellitus;
9. To take care of reduction of other risk factors, e.g. blood pressure; and

10. Public health education; Rising public awareness about diabetes mellitus and its symptoms; Integrating their activity into diabetes mellitus teams; Helping in provision of patient information and education; Checking patient's progress and compliance.

6. COMPLICATIONS

Once upon a time, diabetes was a serious and often fatal disease. Up-to-date, it is still incurable, but it can be effectively managed so as to allow a patient to live a long and near normal life. It is however, a disease that is largely neglected by the general public. This is because the patient do not suffer any pain or major discomfort, seldom dramatically drop dead suddenly and the problem therefore ignored. But the consequence of ignoring the problem can be very serious indeed. It is well known that the disease, if not managed properly, can lead to many other complications. Among these are coronary heart disease, kidney failure, eye problems including blindness, neuropathy and impaired circulation of the feet which could lead to gangrene development and amputation of the leg. Imagine, just by controlling diabetes many of these problems can be avoided or lessened. The disease therefore deserves greater attention by all of us. The first ten years of the diabetic's life are perhaps the most important and if good control is maintained during this period, most patients can escape severe diabetic complications later.

6.1 It Affects All Vital Organs

Diabetes can affect several vital organs, like blood vessels, nervous system, eyes, heart, kidney and feet. How do feet get affected due to diabetes? The blood vessels develop fat deposits, which affects the blood flow and thus reduces blood supply to limbs. The affected part can therefore easily develop infections, leading to gangrene. Smoking can aggravate this problem. Diabetes also affects the nervous system leading to a loss of sensation in several parts of the body. This condition is known as Diabetic Neuropathy. The symptoms of diabetic neuropathy are numbness and loss of sensation in the feet. The patient may feel that he is walking on cotton wool or on a mattress. Often the legs may feel like a "log of wood." There are instances where the chappals fall off and yet the patient is unaware of this. Some patients have even had their toes nibbled-off by rats while sleeping on the ground at night and they were unaware of it! Other patients complain of pins and needles, pricking sensation, burning of feet or even severe pain in both feet.

Diabetic are also prone to high blood pressure and enlargement of the heart. Left untreated, diabetes could affect the kidneys leading to Diabetic Nephropathy, which is the commonest cause of renal failure today necessitating dialysis and renal transplantation.

Eyes are most commonly affected. Diabetes can affect the back portion of the eyes called as the retina. This is called as Diabetic Retinopathy and is the leading cause of blindness. It has therefore been a policy at MVDSC that every diabetic should have his or her eyes examined right from the very first visit to the center and thereafter at least on an annual basis. This will help prevent blindness due to diabetes.

Diabetes can also affect the sexual function leading to impotency in males. Loss of erection and decreased sexual libido are seen in up to 25-30% of diabetics with over 15 years duration of the disease.

Diabetes is one of the causes of premature heart attacks. Indians have the highest prevalence rate of coronary heart disease in the world. Unfortunately, diabetic patients can have heart attacks even without any of the usual symptoms like chest pain, sweating, etc. because the nerves are affected first. This means that careful check-up of the heart should be done even in the absence of symptoms.

6.2 Take Care of Feet

Of all the patients with diabetes; at least 25% will develop foot problems related to the disease. Diabetic foot conditions develop from a combination of causes including poor circulation and neuropathy. Diabetic Neuropathy can cause insensitivity or a loss of ability to feel pain, heat and cold. Diabetics suffering from neuropathy can develop minor cuts, scrapes, blisters, or pressure sores that they may not be aware of due to the insensitivity. If these minor injuries are left untreated, complications may result and lead to ulceration and possibly even amputation. Neuropathy can also cause deformities such as Bunions, Hammer Toes and Charcot Feet.

It is very important for diabetics to take necessary precautions to prevent all foot-related injuries. Due to the consequences of neuropathy, daily observation of the feet is critical. When a diabetic patient takes necessary preventative foot care measures, it reduces the risks of serious foot conditions. Diabetes often leads to peripheral vascular disease, which inhibits a person's blood circulation. With this condition, there is a narrowing of the arteries that frequently leads to significantly decreased circulation in the lower part of the legs and the feet. Poor circulation contributes to diabetic foot problems by reducing the amount of oxygen and nutrition supplied to the skin and other tissue, therefore causing injuries to heal poorly. Poor circulation can also lead to swelling and dryness of the foot. Preventing foot complications is more critical for the diabetic patient since poor circulation impairs the healing process, and can lead to ulcers, infection and other serious foot conditions.

Footwear and orthotics play an important role in diabetic foot care. Orthotics designed with Plastazote foam, the #1 material for protecting the insensitive diabetic foot, is usually recommended. Plastazote is a material designed to accommodate pressure "hot spots" by conforming to heat and pressure. By customizing to the foot, Plastazote provides the comfort and protection needed in diabetic foot care. Footwear constructed with Plastazote is also recommended frequently for the diabetic patient. Diabetic Footwear should also provide the following protective benefits:

- ❑ High, wide toe box (high and wide space in the toe area).
- ❑ Removable in-soles for fitting flexibility and the option to insert orthotics if necessary.
- ❑ *Rocker Soles*: These soles are designed to reduce

pressure in the areas of the foot most susceptible to pain, most notably the ball-of-the-foot.

- ❑ Firm Heel Counters for support and stability.

If you are a diabetic, you should be particularly alert to any problems you may be having with your feet. It is very important for diabetics with neuropathy to take necessary precautions to prevent injury and keep their feet healthy. If you have diabetes and are experiencing a foot problem, immediately consult with your foot doctor. Proper foot care is especially critical for diabetics because they are prone to foot problems such as:

- ❑ Loss of feeling in their feet.
- ❑ Changes in the shape of their feet.
- ❑ Foot ulcers or sores that do not heal.

Simple daily foot care can prevent serious problems. The following are simple everyday steps that will help prevent serious complications from diabetes:

1. Check Diabetes

Make healthy lifestyle choices to keep your blood sugar close to normal. Work with your health care team to create a diabetes plan that fits your lifestyle characteristics.

2. Check Your Feet

You may have foot problems that you may not be aware of. Check your feet for cuts, sores, red spots, swelling, or infected toenails. Checking your feet should become part of your daily routine. If you have trouble bending over to see your feet, use a plastic mirror to help. You can also ask a family member to help you. Important Reminder Be sure to call your doctor immediately if a cut, sore, blister, or bruise on your foot does not heal after one day.

3. Wash Your Feet

Wash your feet in warm, NOT HOT, water. Do not soak your feet because your skin will get dry. Before bathing or showering, test the water to make sure it is not too hot.

You should use a thermometer or your elbow. Dry your feet well. Be sure to dry between your toes. Use talcum powder to keep the skin dry between the toes.

4. Keep the Skin Soft and Smooth

Rub a thin coat of skin lotion or crème on the tops and bottoms of the feet. Do not put lotion between your toes, because this might cause infection.

5. Trim Your Toenails Each Week

Trim your toenails with clippers after you wash and dry your feet. Trim the toenails straight across and smooth them with emery board or nail file. DO NOT cut into the corners of the nail or rip-off hangnails. If your nails are thick or yellowed, DO NOT cut your own nails, have a foot doctor trim them.

6. Wear Shoes and Socks

Wear shoes and socks at all times. Do not walk barefoot, not even indoors. It is extremely easy to step on something and hurt your feet. Always wear seamless socks, stockings, and nylons with your shoes to help avoid the possibility of blisters and sores developing. Be sure to choose seamless socks that are made of materials that wick moisture away from your feet and absorb shock and shear. Socks made of these materials help keep your feet dry. Always check the insides of your shoes before putting them on. Make sure the lining is smooth and there are no foreign objects in the shoe, such as pebbles. Wear shoes that fit well and protect your feet.

7. Protect Your Feet From Hot and Cold

Always wear shoes. Put sunscreen on the tops of your feet for protection from the sun. Keep your feet away from radiators or open fires. DO NOT use hot water bottle or heating pads on your feet. If your feet are cold, wear seamless socks at night. Lined boots are good to keep your feet warm in the winter. Choose socks carefully. DO NOT wear socks with seams or bumpy areas. Choose padded socks to protect your feet and make walking more comfortable. In cold weather, check your feet often to keep your feet warm avoid frostbite.

- ❑ Keep the Blood Flowing to your Feet. Put your feet up when you are sitting. Wiggle your toes for 5 minutes, 2 or 3 times a day. Move your ankles up and down and in and out to improve blood flow in your feet and legs. DO NOT cross your legs for long periods of time.
- ❑ DO NOT wear tight socks, elastic, or rubber bands, or garters around your legs.
- ❑ DO NOT wear restrictive footwear or foot products. Diabetics should not wear foot products that can cut-off circulation to the feet, such as products with elastic.
- ❑ DO NOT smoke. Smoking reduces blood flow to your feet.

If you have high blood pressure or high cholesterol, work with your health care team to lower it.

Be More Active

Ask your doctor to plan an exercise program that is right for you. Walking, dancing, swimming, and bicycling are good forms of exercise that are easy on the feet. Avoid all activities that are hard on the feet, such as running and jumping. Always include a short warm-up or cool-down period. Wear protective walking or athletic shoes that fit well and offer good support. Ask your doctor to check the sense of feeling and pulses in your feet at least once a year. Ask your doctor to tell you immediately if you have serious foot problems.

- ❑ If you are 45 or over, you should be tested every three years.
- ❑ You should be tested earlier and more frequently if you:
  - Are obese (more than 20% above healthy body weight). The obesity rate has risen dramatically during the past two decades and

now includes one-third of Americans.
- Have a parent or sibling with diabetes.
- Is black, or belong to another high-risk ethnic group, e.g. Indian.
- Gave birth to a baby weighing more than nine pounds, or developed gestational diabetes during pregnancy.
- Have high blood pressure (140/90 or higher).
- Have an HDL ("good") cholesterol level of 35 or below and/or a blood triglyceride level of 250 or higher.

❑ 126 mg/dl (milligrams of glucose in one-tenth liter of blood) or more, on a fasting stomach, means you have diabetes.

Blood Sugar (mg/dl)	*Diagnosis*
Less than 110	Normal
110-125	Impaired fasting glucose
126 and above (twice)	Diabetes

❑ If you are diagnosed with diabetes in its early stages, you'll be advised to lose weight if you're overweight, exercise more, improve your diet (choose the same low-fat, semi-vegetarian diet that is known to lower the risk of heart disease and cancer), and quit smoking if you smoke. The goal of early detection is to avoid diabetes medications, or at least postpone or minimize their use, not merely to start drug therapy earlier.

❑ If your result is between 110 and 125, you fall into a new category called "impaired fasting glucose," a danger zone or borderline area. This means that you should take the same steps as outlined above, since blood sugar levels tend to rise with age. Here is where it may truly be possible to prevent diabetes.

7. DIABETES PREVENTION

7.1 Strike at Pre-diabetes

1 out of 3 Americans (Indians are fast catching in

obesity) have a condition called insulin resistance syndrome, also called metabolic syndrome or syndrome X. It refers to people whose bodies don't manage insulin well. More people are developing the condition as the population eats more and exercises less, and it puts them at high risk of diabetes and heart disease. If not dealt with it can also develop into fatty liver, colon or ovarian cancer. Even 7-10 year old children are developing this condition. There is no one single test to determine this syndrome, but measurements combining weight, blood pressure, cholesterol and glucose tolerance can. A simple home test is waist circumference. Men with 40-inch and women with 35-inch waist circumference are at high risk. This syndrome could be remedied by more exercise and less food intake. In addition, this stunning revelation puts also the welfare of the whole population at risk. "It is inconceivable that our nation can have the resources to deal with 100 million potential diabetics and heart condition victims. If we don't deal with it now, we will bankrupt our economy", said one American study. It is equally well applicable to Indians.

Persons with impaired glucose tolerance (IGT) have a high risk of developing Type 2 diabetes. In a study in China it was demonstrated that, lifestyle intervention over 6 years led to a significant decrease in incidence of Type 2 diabetes. Several exercise intervention studies have concluded that physical activity interventions might be successful in a community setting. As the majority of cases of Type 2 diabetes appear to be related to lifestyle, Type 2 diabetes could be seen as an exercise deficiency or dietary excess disorder, and is potentially preventable through the pursuit of a healthy way of life. This is a landmark study. The development of IGT to Type 2 diabetes was reduced by a third in the intervention groups compared with controls. The effect of diet was similar to that of exercise.

7.2 Yoga is Useful

Yoga claims to be beneficial for many diseases and problems. But there is generally a lack of research, which shows that yoga can actually help in certain diseases. Even the few studies which have been done have not been sufficient in the public eye, and there is a need to highlight what the studies are showing about how different systems can help in different situations The Yoga Institute, Santa Cruz has been actively involved in studying the actual effects of yoga. Since 1987 they have been holding camps for people with particular types of ailments and actually keeping records on how their advice, exercise regimes, diet advice helps in the ailment. These short-term 2-day camps, which give a holistic approach, have had a great effect on those who participated. The Yoga Institute emphasizes a change in values through changed attitudes and new habits culminating in a new healthy lifestyle as the management technique in diabetes. The Yoga Plan for Total Health is a carefully conceived training program, which includes:

(i) Helping to establish healthy routines through change in diet, sleep and posture.
(ii) Self-care through urine testing.
(iii) Understanding the emotional implications of the disease and how to overcome anxiety and apathy, and the consequent swings in blood sugar levels.
(iv) How to eat, what to eat, when to eat and why not to eat certain foods.
(v) Exercising and stretching the spine and various muscles of the body through yogic practice.
(vi) Yogic breathing and concentration through Asanas, Pranayamas, Kriyas such as Trataka, Candle Gazing, Jalneti and Kapalbhati.
(vii) Yogic relaxation mainly Savasana, Nispandbhava and Dradhasana as destressors.
(viii) Acceptance of Yogic Philosophy and way of life, with group discussions, sharing sessions and Karma Yoga.
(ix) A period of Maunavrat (silence) for stock-taking and reflection, and Abhyasa to put learning into practice.

Follow-ups revealed that those who kept up their practice and changed their basic attitudes towards life show a marked and consistent improvement in their DM status. The results of 40 patients who attended a camp were studied.

The age group was 30-68 years, and there were 32 males and 8 females. Most of them were non-insulin depended patients with average duration of diabetes ranging from 3-5 years. At the beginning of the study, blood sugar was tested. After the camp, the blood sugar, urine sugar, weight and blood sugar were tested again. The tests showed that both fasting and PP blood sugar showed a distinct fall to near normal values, requiring significant reduction in medicines.

7.3 The Screening Test

New guidelines lower the cut-off points between normal, borderline, and high (diabetic) levels of blood sugar. That, combined with widespread screening, is expected to identify additional cases of diabetics. And the half that have been diagnosed typically have the disease for seven years before it is diagnosed. Experts hope that early detection will identify cases when they are still mild. It's hoped that this way, before symptoms develop, people can take steps to minimize the subtle damage to organs and blood vessels caused by years of high blood sugar levels, and avoid later complications of diabetes, such as heart disease, hypertension, stroke, and diseases of the eyes, nerves, and kidneys, which often lead to premature death.

7.4 The Diet

Many people still believe that eating too much sugar causes diabetes. This misconception arises because diabetes is diagnosed by measuring blood sugar/glucose. But dietary sugar is only a part of the picture. A diet rich in certain high-carbohydrate foods—those low in fiber and with a high glycemic index (GI)-increases the risk of Type 2 diabetes, at least in those predisposed to it. One study tracked 65,000 female nurses (age 40 to 65); the other followed 43,000 male health professionals. Over the course of six years, a total of 1,438 developed diabetes. Men and women whose diet had a high glycemic index and low fiber content more than doubled their chance of developing diabetes. Foods that seemed to pose the greatest risk were white bread, white rice, potatoes, and sugary soft drinks. In contrast, whole-grain breads and cereals (rich in fiber and with a lower glycemic index) appeared to reduce the risk of diabetes. The researchers suggested that excessive amounts of carbohydrate-rich foods with a high glycemic index put pressure on the pancreas to produce more of the hormone insulin, which stimulates the body's cells to take in and store glucose. Over time, the body may become resistant to insulin. In such insulin-resistant people, the cells become less and less sensitive to insulin. This is characteristic of Type 2 diabetes. Of course, not everyone on such a low-fiber, high-starch diet develops diabetes. There seems to be a genetic predisposition to diabetes, which may be exacerbated by this kind of diet. Obesity is probably the leading risk factor for Type 2 diabetes. Family history of the disease, advancing age, and lack of exercise are other important factors.

7.5 Magnesium has a Role

A study found that the mineral magnesium has a protective effect against diabetes. A few studies have suggested that this mineral improves insulin sensitivity. But since whole grains are rich in magnesium, it's hard to say whether the proposed benefit is due to something else in the grain (notably its fiber) or the mineral.

Bottom line: A diabetes-prevention diet, if there is one, is the same low-fat, high-fiber, semi-vegetarian diet that is known to lower the risk of heart disease and cancer. The Harvard studies simply underline the importance of choosing whole-grain products, as opposed to highly refined, low-fiber grain products such as white bread, in order to help control blood sugar. Such a diet helps in weight control. It also provides the vitamins, minerals, and other nutrients you need to help prevent chronic diseases, including, perhaps, diabetes.

7.6 The Glycemic Index (GI)

The glycemic index indicates how fast a high-carbohydrate food is digested into glucose and how much it causes blood glucose to rise. The index doesn't depend merely on whether the carbohydrates are simple (sugars) or complex (starches). Many factors come into play, including the amount of fiber and fat in the food, how refined the food is, how fast the food is digested, whether it was cooked, and what else is eaten with it. Table sugar and honey have a high glycemic index (meaning they have a strong effect on blood sugar). But so do raisins, corn, potatoes, carrots, white bread, instant rice, and most refined cereals. Though sweet, apples and peaches, as well as beans, grapefruit, and peanuts, have a low glycemic index. Pasta gets a middle rating, as does oatmeal. There is no reason to avoid foods with a high glycemic index—many are very nutritious. Even people predisposed to diabetes, or with the disease, can eat these foods in moderation:

1. If you're over 45, get a fasting plasma glucose test every three years.
2. Keep your weight under control. Stay close to the ideal weight for your height, age and gender.
3. Eat low-fat, low-sugar meals rich in vegetables and whole grain foods.
4. Exercise enough to sweat at least 30 minutes 3 to 4 times a week. This indicates cardiovascular benefits.
5. Take effective steps to lower high blood pressure.
6. Achieve healthy levels of cholesterol and triglycerides.
7. Stop smoking.

Better nutrition, physical activity, control of blood glucose levels, and access to services can delay the progression of diabetes. In fact, recent findings show that modest, consistent physical activity and a healthy diet can cut a person's risk for developing Type 2 diabetes by nearly 60 percent.

8. WOMEN HAVE TO CARE EXTRA

Diabetes adds to your problems, if you are in the menopausal zone, esp. your heart is greatly endangered.

With all the headlines about the dangers of hormone replacement therapy, I am confused. I am a 60-year-old, healthy woman who began taking hormone replacements because I was sick of the hot flashes, night sweats and mood swings I was experiencing while I was going through menopause. Can you give me some information on the pros and cons of taking these drugs? I don't know if I should throw in the towel and use it to wipe my brow during hot flashes or keep taking my estrogen? Before menopause sets in your heart is supposed to be protected by your female hormones, but not after menopause. However, if you have diabetes, the heart is unprotected even before the menopause has set in. Hormone replacement therapy includes either estrogen or a combination of estrogen/progestin, available only by prescription. Menopause is the transition between a woman's child-bearing and non-child-bearing years. It is the last stage of the biological process during which the ovaries gradually produce lower levels of estrogen, progesterone and testosterone. A natural occurrence much like puberty, menopause causes a variety of reactions in the body including hot flashes, night sweats, sleeplessness, loss of bone density and vaginal dryness. However, use of hormone replacement therapy at the appropriate time and under supervision of your gynecologist is a good proposition. Medical professionals say hormone replacement therapy still has its place and could be an option for the right reasons at the right times. However, ·it appears long-term hormone replacement usage might not be advisable. Furthermore, menopause occurs at mid-life, a time when many women already are overstressed with teenage children, aging parents and full-time jobs. These factors could contribute to the symptoms of menopause. There are plenty of natural remedies for women to use to help endure the effects of menopause and stay healthy through the aging process. Among them are: exercise for the heart; lifting weights and drinking milk to combat osteoporosis; beefing up on veggies and regular colon check-ups; keeping blood pressure down to prevent strokes.

9. FAQS

Here are some frequently asked questions:

Q. What is the role of exercise in the prevention and treatment of DM?

Only a small fraction of Indians moderately exercise on a regular basis. It was estimated for American population, that inactivity contributed to 32% of all cases of heart disease; 18% of all cases of high blood pressure; 32% of all strokes; 18% of all diabetes; and 23% of all cases of osteoporosis. Indian figures would be much higher. Diabetes is the leading cause of blindness, kidney disease, amputations and retinopathy. The American Diabetes Prevention Program demonstrated that individuals who had impaired glucose tolerance, but who did not yet have diabetes, could reduce their risk for developing diabetes by losing 5-7% of their excess body weight and being moderately active for 30 minutes a day. The Diabetes Control and Complication Trial showed improved blood glucose control in those with Type 1 diabetes reduces diabetic neuropathy by 60%, retinopathy by 34%, and kidney disease by 56%.

It would be a good habit to start using artificial sweeteners in cooking, eating at least 3 vegetables and 2 fruits a day, using reduced or non-fat products, eating more fish and seafood, and using salt substitutes in cooking. Do we "eat to live" or "live to eat"? For most of us, the first is true, as one must eat to live. But there may be times when the enjoyment of food is more important to you than the nourishment you get from it. When a person is initially diagnosed with diabetes mellitus, the mind turns to diet first. Will I have to give up my favourite foods? Am I facing a lifetime of bland, salt free and sugar free meals? The answer fortunately is 'no' and you don't have to follow some kind of special "Diabetic diet." All one has to do is to eat a "Balanced" meal plan that is required to lead a healthy life.

Normally the body produces a hormone called insulin. In people with diabetes, the ability to make or utilize insulin is impaired. Without Insulin, the body cannot absorb or use glucose, the simple sugar the body produces from the food that we eat. Insulin is the key that unlocks the cells and lets the glucose enter, where it is oxidized to yield energy for all life activities. Diet has always had a key role to play in the management of diabetes. In fact, until insulin became available, 'Special' diets were the only form of treatment. The term 'Diet' does not mean that one has to eat monotonous and restricted foods. Nor does it mean that one has to give up the food one enjoys. Instead, the goal is to develop a healthy "eating style" that will help you combat diabetes as well as contribute to improving overall health.

Q. Can People with Diabetes eat normal food?

There's no such thing as a diabetic diet. A diabetic individual can eat the same food as the rest of the family members with a few modifications to have good glycemic control. Healthy foods don't raise blood sugar. Even nutritious food like whole wheat bread, fruit and oatmeal can raise blood sugar to an unhealthy level. The balance between insulin and carbohydrate is what determines blood sugar control, not whether the food is packed with vitamins and minerals or not. To control diabetes you need to know how to manage carbohydrates whether they come from nutritious food you eat everyday or from sweets you eat less often.

Q. Does the intakc of Sugar causes diabetes?

When sugar is consumed, the hormone insulin is required to bring blood glucose level normal. Diabetes is caused due to a lack of insulin, not due to excess of sugar in the diet. Once someone has diabetes, it is important to manage the frequency and the amount of eating and the type of carbohydrates (simple or complex) including sugar consumed to allow the body to maintain good blood sugar control. Sugars are better avoided as they contribute nothing other than calories and also have a high glycemic index. However, simply eating sugar does not produce diabetes.

Q. The consumption of neem and bitter gourd at regular intervals cures diabetes. True?

This is the widespread myth and quite a large number of people subscribe to it. Unfortunately, there very light truth in it. Nevertheless, neem and bitter gourd, because of their pronounced bitter taste, may deactivate the taste buds, for short spells, thus lessening the total food intake. Also, they do have some blood sugar lowering properties but they do certainly do not 'cure' diabetes.

Q. Can the People with diabetes eat as much of sugar free products as they want or foods labeled 'diabetic' or 'suitable for people with diabetes'?

Many sugar free products contain calories. Read the label carefully. Remember that "natural" does not necessarily mean "safe." It not necessary for anyone with diabetic to eat 'special diabetic' foods. Most products consist of a range of confectionery foods sweetened with a sweetener like sorbitol or fructose, instead of ordinary sugar. They tend to be just as high in fat and calories as their non-diabetic counterparts and may also cost more money.

Q. Diabetics can eat wheat but not rice. True or false?

This is not true. Both wheat and rice have the same amount of carbohydrate (~70%) and have almost similar glycemic index and raise the blood sugar to a similar extent. Therefore, it should not matter whether one takes wheat or rice as long as the total quantity is restricted.

Q. Can you suggest a meal plan?

The proportion of carbohydrate, protein and fat in our eating plan depends on weight, glycemic control, blood cholesterol level, and medical needs. What we eat depends on what foods we enjoy. The wide variety of foods may offer a healthy way of eating that's good for the whole family. A minimum of three meals should consume eaten per day. Ideally they should be evenly sized, evenly spaced and should more or less at the same time of day every day. All meals and snacks should preferably contain a source of carbohydrate. Food intake must correlate with the duration of peak action of the medication to maintain euglycaemia at all times. The type and time of medication administration and the timing of the last meal determine the need for the in between snack. The specifics of diabetic meal planning need to be designed with the individual's needs in mind. This is where a dietitian specializing in diabetes comes in as she can educate about the portion sizes, meal composition, and timing of meals or snacks. Meal plans are custom-designed based on patients' tastes, preferences, and lifestyle. They must also meet the patients' diabetes goals and nutritional requirements.

Skipping meals or eating at different times each day can make it difficult to keep the blood sugar level under control. Skipping meals often makes one too hungry at time of the next meal and thus one tends to eat more. One should therefore try to eat at regular meal timings and stick to it as far as possible. Matching food to insulin peak helps you to achieve control of blood sugar. Patients with Type I diabetes mellitus must understand the action of particular meal and snacks to avoid low blood sugar. Type II Diabetic patients may have to switch from three standard meals to three lighter meals interspaced with snacks throughout the day if necessary. A diet plan for a pregnant woman who has diabetes should be based on a nutritional assessment. This is true whether her diabetes is pre-existing or whether she has gestational diabetes. A dietitian can help to create and adjust a meal plan based on the needs of both mother and baby's blood glucose levels—

- Dietary management should form part of the total lifestyle management of a person, and is considered to be the backbone of the management of diabetes. The broad objectives for the dietary management are: To achieve optimal glucose concentrations.
- To achieve optimal lipid concentrations.
- To provide appropriate energy for reasonable weight, normal growth and development and, pregnancy and lactation.
- To prevent, delay and treat nutrition-related complications.

Q What is optimal nutrition for cases of DM?

To improve health through optimal nutrition. A low-fat, low-cholesterol diet is recommended because people with diabetes are at greater risk for heart disease than the general population. Where the carbohydrate content is already high, e.g. in India, items like potatos, bread, pasta must be reduced or substituted for rice or wheat. The healthiest choices are ones that contain vitamins, minerals, and fiber, such as whole grains. Carbohydrates need to be spread out throughout the day, not eaten all at once at one large meal. Complex carbohydrate is preferred to simple carbohydrates. Many factors can influence one's blood glucose levels, including the size of a meal, the fat or fiber content, eating slowly, and the amount and type of medication taken, if any. Increase intake of vegetable protein (15-20% of calorie intake) and dietary fiber (40-50 g/day). Overall dietary recommendations for diabetes are similar to those for the general healthy population: eat a diet rich in fruits, veggies, and whole grains, with moderate amounts of lean proteins and non-fat or low-fat dairy, and small amounts of fats and oils, mostly from monounsaturated sources, such as olive and canola oils.

Q. How the carbohydrates affect DM?

Learn about the carbohydrate in foods and how they affect your diabetes. This knowledge will give you power and freedom. The old saying: "Prevention is better than cure", is very true when it comes to diabetes, because it is a life-long condition for which there is no cure. By living a healthy lifestyle, a person whether he/she is vulnerable or not can prevent the onset of diabetes and by careful control, a person with diabetes may avoid the severe complications and lead a full and normal life. Eat meals and prescribed snacks at regular times each day. Avoid food, high in sugar content such as honey, jellies, candy, syrup and soft drinks. Certain fruits like papaya, small plantain, apple, etc. can be taken, provided your blood sugar is under control. Avoid fruits with high sugar content like mango, jackfruit, sapota, etc.

- Eat cereals like rice in limited quantities and increase vegetable content of meals.
- Do not skip meals or prescribed snacks. This is

particularly important in those taking insulin injection.

- Regular daily exercise plays an important part in diabetes control. Exercise helps to: Utilize glucose effectively, which reduces the amount of insulin needed. Reduce weight; weight loss can improve your diabetes. Regular exercise program can prevent cardiovascular complications. Exercise relieves stress and tension and a well-exercised body feels good. The three key aspects in any exercise program are: Frequency, Intensity and Timing. Exercise should be done frequently, i.e. at least 5 times a week. It should be intense. Exercise should be intense enough to burn sufficient calories. Timing: Minimum 45 minutes to one hour walking is important for getting maximum benefit. A very common misconception about insulin is that once insulin is started, it has to be taken lifelong. This is not always true. Many patients with Type 2 diabetes require insulin treatment for a short period only. The following circumstances warrant insulin treatment when the blood sugar levels are very high, the chances of tablets working are less because of a condition called glucose toxicity. In this situation, if insulin treatment is started, blood sugar levels can be brought back to normal and then patients can be switched over to tablets.

Q. When is insulin required?

It is required in certain special situation like prior to and during surgery, in case of any serious infections, during emergencies like heart attacks, and during pregnancy. When tablets should not be taken. After this period one can resume tablets again. If your diabetes is being treated with insulin or oral medication, you may occasionally have symptoms of hypoglycemia (or low blood sugar). This might occur, if you ate less than usual, or missed meals altogether. Unusual amounts of exercise can also cause the blood sugars to dip. Common symptoms of hypoglycemia include drowsiness, headache, slurred speech, confusion, excessive sweating, hunger and pounding of the heart. If hypoglycemia occurs at night, patient may experience difficulty in sleeping, nightmares or an early morning headache. Hypoglycemia should be promptly recognized and treated, as otherwise the patient can go on to a stage of coma. Mild hypoglycemia can be managed by taking coffee with sugar a chocolate or even a snack. If it is not responding to these measures, the patient should be taken to a doctor or given glucose injections through a vein. Diabetic patients should always carry a card, which gives details regarding his or her disease and treatment so that hypoglycemia can be easily recognized and treated.

Q. What is the role of repeated blood testing?

Continued blood sugar testing, by both you and your doctor, is essential in treating diabetes. The purpose of routine testing is to see how your treatment program is working and to see whether any changes should be made or not. You can test either a drop of blood from your fingertip or use urine samples. Testing blood is more accurate and may allow better control of your sugar levels. Testing glucose levels in the blood serves as useful check on diabetes and it also keeps you motivated to control your blood sugar better. Blood sugar testing at home using a blood glucose meter has now become easier and more convenient. If you cannot afford this, the next best is to urine sugar testing either with Benedicts solution or a test strip—the latter is easier and less messy. Early in the treatment, you may have to test daily, even twice or thrice a day. Later when the blood sugar has stabilized testing weekly twice would be sufficient. Tests can be done one day in the morning, next time after lunch and the next time after dinner. Not only is testing important, but you should also keep a chart of your sugar levels, which will be useful to your doctor to adjust your medication. Glycosylated hemoglobin is a relatively new blood test that will give you the average blood sugar levels over the past 2-3 months. This test has become the "gold standard" in the management of diabetes. Both the doctor and the patient should strive to bring Hba1c as close to 7%, which is the value termed as good control. Good control will go a long way in preventing diabetic complications. Glucowatch: This is a new device to test your blood sugar levels even without pricking! This is still in the trial stage and is presently quite expensive.

Q. What are different kinds of insulins?

- *Newer insulin*: Newer and faster acting insulin called insulin analogues have come which provides flexibility to the patient in relation to timing the meals.
- *Pancreas transplantation*: Improvements in pancreas and islet transplantation provide a great hope for Type 1 diabetic patients for achieving a total cure of diabetes.
- *Nasal insulin*: Newer insulin delivery devices include nasal sprays, which need not be injected. This insulin treatment is in the final stages of development.

Newer drugs: Newer oral drugs are now becoming available which will help in reducing blood sugar levels better and more efficiently than existing compounds.

Q. Can diabetes be prevented?

Yes. Diabetes can be prevented from developing in a susceptible person like those with a strong family history and those who are obese. Diet, exercise, weight reduction and stress management can achieve this.

Q. My father has Type I diabetes, and I have high concerns about the genetic inheritance of this disease. I am 23 and keep a pretty healthy diet involving much produce, juices, fish, and proteins. (I must confess I have a sweet tooth as well.). From my understanding, the inheritance of diabetes is due to both genetics and the environment. Are there preventative measures that I can take or is it a fact if I am going to inherit diabetes?

Based on genetics studies, there's a small chance (about

5 to 10%) that you will develop Type 1 diabetes. Simple blood test for the presence of antibodies against the insulin-making cells is required. There's nothing you can do to alter the genetic odds. As for the environmental component, it is possible that your current healthy lifestyle may decrease the likelihood that you will develop diabetes. We always encourage family members, as well as our patients, to maintain a healthy diet, physical activity, and a positive outlook on life.

3

Learn Proper Posture and Proper Walking: Two Keys to Total Fitness

RAVINDER SINGH AND JASMINE SACHDEVA

Body posture is the relative position of various parts of body in relation to each other. Basically, it is body alignment with respect to ever-present force of gravity. Whether we are standing, sitting or lying down, gravity exerts force on our joints, ligaments, muscles and other parts of body. Good posture entails distributing the force of gravity through our body so that no structure is over stressed.

Human body is like a well-constructed building and has to withstand same type of stresses and strains. As a building with poor foundation, a body with poor posture is less resistant to stresses and strains of life.

Man is different from other animals for the fact that he has assumed an erect posture. Where other animals walk on four limbs, man walks on hind limbs (legs) with fore limbs (arms) hanging by the side. This evolutionary erect posture of man has resulted in remarkable flexibility and mobility of body at the expenses of stability, thus putting extra strain on

* Professor & Head, Department of Orthopedics, Government Medical College, Patiala.

various body parts.

Posture is just natural and a part of habit. It is constantly changing. Different acts of daily living require different posture. Whether sleeping, sitting, standing, walking, running or doing any other work, one requires a definite and a different posture. Different body postures put different amount of stress on various parts of body. Of course, there can be good postures and bad postures.

Good posture is elegant and noted by others, raises self-esteem and confidence of a person, is energy efficient and is useful in maintaining a healthy lifestyle. It allows one to work longer and play longer.

On the other hand, bad posture is a sign of unhealthy living, wastes energy and may result in chronic fatigue, headache, backache, lethargy, muscular strain, etc.

Backache, which is one of the most common health complaint and wastes more man-hours than any other work-related problem is mostly because of a bad work posture. Postural stress due to habitually incorrect posture like prolonged sitting in poor position, prolonged bending in bad work position, incorrect lifting of heavy weights or standing and lying down in poor position strains the ligaments leading to chronic back pain. Over the period of time uncorrected habitually poor posture causes structural changes in the joints, with increased wear and tear. Thus, long-term effects of poor posture can be as severe and as bad as an injury. In some cases even surgery may be required to correct the defect or to prevent deterioration. (See Appendix II, 'Disc Surgery' for more details).

Some natural postures of daily activity are being described in the following passages for the awareness of the readers.

SLEEPING

Lying down and sleeping is the most basic posture of man. It gives rest to the body, relieves stress, removes fatigue and re-energizes man for work. On average a person spends 1/3 of his lifetime in sleep. Thus, a good sleeping habit and posture are absolutely essential.

First of all, we should sleep on a bed which is large enough to permit movements during sleep, firm enough to support without sagging. It should be neither too hard nor too soft. It should be soft enough on the top to accommodate contours of the spine. Sleeping on your back, use a pillow to keep you head in a neutral position, neither too high nor too low. Straight-backed people will need thinner pillow than rounded shoulder people. Pillow should be a feather/cotton fiber filled, that shapes itself to the contour of the neck. Even a soft foam pillow can do. A too firm or too bulky pillow does not fulfil the postural needs and can be a cause of headaches as well as neck and upper back discomfort. Patients of cervical or neck pains can do well with contoured orthopaedic pillows easily available at medical stores. Sleep on the side or back. Do not sleep on stomach as it is unnatural for the back and also forcibly turns the head to one side straining the neck.

Generally, when sleeping on the side, thickness of the pillow should be equal to the space between the neck and shoulders and will vary from person to person depending upon the body structure. When sleeping on the back it is advantageous to keep a small support under the neck.

Correct sleeping position allows one to sleep comfortably and to wake up without increased pain or discomfort. Although people change position while sleeping, they can begin a night's rest according to some general guidelines, which will increase comfort. Avoid sleeping on couches or chairs. Only the bed can provide the freedom of movement needed to avoid unnecessary back strain. Couches and chairs are also more prone to sag and most chairs don't support the neck.

While sleeping on the back one can keep a pillow under the knees if desired. While sleeping on the side it is comfortable to keep the lower leg fairly straight with upper leg bent at the hip and knee with a pillow between the knees.

Persons having lung or chest disease require head and chest to be elevated. Consider raising the head of the bed.

One should not abruptly lie flat or sit up suddenly. For lying down sit on the sides of the bed, gently recline sideways being careful to use your arm nearest to the head side of the bed for support, swaying your legs (still bent) up in the bed and now you will be lying on you side, straighten the legs and turn. You are comfortably lying on you back. To get out of the bed reverse the process. Turn to the side, flex the hips and knees with the support of the arm reclining, get up bringing your legs down and sit up.

To get up from the bed slide up to the edge of the bed, plant feet firmly on the floor directly under you, place your hands on your bed on the sides or on your thighs and push you're hands down to lift up the body and straighten up.

SITTING

As one sits the pelvis rotates and the lower back straightens. Sit tall with both feet on the floor and your whole back against the chair with head erect; the body weight should be evenly distributed. The back should be comfortably supported. Use arm rests if available.

Avoid hunching forward, if using a stool, place it close to your work surface so as to rest your arms comfortably, also use the height adjustment if available to assure comfortable positioning. Sitting position is where most of us get into trouble with poor posture habits. This is especially true when driving or using a computer. As we focus on the activity in front of use, we tend to protrude head and neck forwards. Because the body follows the head, thoracic and lumber spine tend to round forwards as well. When this occurs the weight of the head and upper body is no longer balanced over the spinal column but instead must be supported by increased muscular energy and placing spinal ligaments on stretch, over times, this leads to fatigue and eventually pain in the neck and upper back. Forward rounding of shoulders commonly occurs when car seat is too far away from the steering.

Ideally the S-shaped curvature of the spine, which is characteristic of good standing posture, should be maintained in sitting as well. This is best accomplished by sitting all the way back in a straight backed chair and placing a folded towel or small pillow in the area of the low back. Many new office chairs and car seats come with built in lumbar support and other adjustable features.

STANDING

When we look at some one's posture we generally first look at the alignment of weight bearing joints in standing. Ideally viewed from the back, the spine should have no side curvature or tilt and the legs should be symmetrical without undue angulations at the knees or ankles. From a side view the spine should form a smooth S-shaped curve bisected by an imaginary plum line dropped from the apex of the head. With this alignment the body weight is balanced requiring minimal muscular efforts and avoiding excessive stress on ligaments.

When standing, your lower back should curve slightly forwards. This curve is called lumbar lordosis and helps to transmit weight through the spine and pelvis.

Stand tall; knees should be straight but not locked, stomach flat, ribs raised, shoulders and head erect. Pretend you are balancing an object on your head. Your weight should be evenly distributed on both the legs.

Sitting and standing with proper postural alignment will allow one to work more efficiently with less fatigue and strain of body ligaments and muscles.

WALKING

Walk tall with your feet pointing straight ahead. Arms should swing freely from the sides. Look straight ahead and never down.

To improve gait draw a straight line, keep a full-length mirror at the distant end and walk on the straight line only. The distance between the steps must be equal all the time, look straight into the mirror and walk with a steady pace.

RUNNING

Millions of people over the world are jogging and running as a part of daily exercise programme. Up to 70% of them at some time will sustain a running related injury due to some fault in the surface, shoe, posture, technique or training. Injuries are most common when runners begin a running programme or progress from one level to another. Beginning runners, enthusiastic and out of shape are often hurt when they run too much, too soon or run on hard surfaces wearing poorly made or inappropriate shoes.

More experienced runners incur over use or stress injuries when they increase their mileage too quickly and run many competitive races or simply over load the musculo skeletal system when training for competitions.

For running a proper running surface is essential. A soft level dirt part is ideal. Running on concrete side walks and up and down curbs exaggerate the shock transmitted to the legs, feet and back. Asphalt roads; on the other hand, provide more cushioning. Grassy surfaces are irregular and sand is unstable. A sloping or banked surface, such as a beach or a shoulder of road forces the foot on the higher part of the slope, putting additional stress on the tendons and ligaments of hind limbs. Up hill running strains heel tendon and muscles of lower back, down hill running increases impact at heel strike.

Poorly constructed or worn out shoes or inappropriate shoes such as sneakers can also contribute to injury because they lack necessary cushioning or stability to protect the foot and leg from repetitive shocks of running.

Running gait consists of a sequence of support and air born (non-support) phases. During running feet collide with the ground 50-70 times per minute, for each foot at a force 2-4 times the body weight. The impact is absorbed by the running shoes or transmitted directly to the legs and the back. Thus, a minor fault in running technique or minor defect in shoe or running surface can have profound effect during running.

For running properly one requires an upright relaxed posture with the trunk perpendicular to the running surface. The upper body neck and arms should be relaxed, the elbows flexed to an angle of 90 to 100 degrees and the hands held loosely. Flexing the elbows to 45 to 50 degrees and clenching the fists can cause pain in the shoulder and pectoral muscles.

Increased arm swing in uphill running improves forward propulsion.

Essential factors in prevention of running injuries are appropriate proper running surface, good quality running shoes, appropriate level of training, and warm up, e.g. exercises performed in preparation of running.

WORK

Incorrect posture at work is the commonest cause of back pain the world over. Habitually incorrect posture like prolonged sitting in poor position, prolonged bending in bad work position, incorrect lifting of heavy weights, standing or lying in improper position at work can strain ligaments and muscles and be a cause of chronic backache. Faulty design of transport for commercial and office seating contributes to poor posture work habits. For example, most chairs hardly provide adequate supports to the lower back. Thus, unless people make conscious effort to sit correctly they are faced with prospects of having to cope with a lifetime low backache. Mere availability of friendly furniture is not enough, the user must be aware of correct back care practices. An informed user can lessen the impact of even poorly designed furniture at work. Prolonged work in same posture whether standing or sitting causes discomfort to spine and it is advisable to take short breaks and incorporate movements to counteract discomfort and fatigue. A well-designed work place has a direct impact on employee's comfort, job satisfaction motivation, sense and well-being and accomplishment.

While at Work

- ❑ Avoid using straight back chairs with no low back support.
- ❑ Ensure that feet are flat on the floor or the footrest.
- ❑ Ensure that your lumbar region is properly protected when seated.
- ❑ Use head rests if your head tilts forwards or backwards for prolonged period. The head is

relatively heavy if not kept straight the pull of gravity will cause stress and strain of muscles of the neck.

Desk Height

- Desk height should be at level with your elbows when the forearms are parallel to the floor. If the desk is too low, raise it with desk raisers if too high then use floor rest and raise your height accordingly. Use inclined plane on the desk for comfort at work.
- While at work take regular breaks from work to do simple stretching exercises for at last one minute every hour.
- Sit up straight in a chair that supports your lower back. While using a keyboard adjust your seat height so that your forearms are horizontal and your elbows at right angles. Vary your tasks so that you are not making the same movements for hours. Tilt your seat forward; if possible, and then adjust your seat so that your chair back is supportive and correctly adjusted in this position.

Computer Screen

- Position should be at arms length and adjust for height so that the tip of your nose is reflected centrally on the screen when correctly seated. Position the screen at 90 degree to any strong light source especially daylight and alter screen angle to avoid glare or reflection. Use a copyholder to keep your input data within your natural field of view. Avoid staying in same position for hours on. Stand up and stretch every 20-30 minutes. If your chair has a free float facility, use it regularly.
- While driving, move the seat for enough forward to allow knees and elbows to be slightly bent as you reach the steering wheel and pedals. Use

added low back support.

- Avoid slouching while driving, or putting the seat too forwards or backwards.
- When lifting heavy objects squat, lift the object close to your body and lift with your thighs keeping the back straight.

Exercise

- Exercise is the key to healthy living. It tones up the muscles and internal organs. Increases flow of blood, improve oxygenation of tissues, corrects body metabolism and removes the toxic matter.
- Exercise is an essential ingredient of any health programme. Stretching and strengthening exercise (warm up) should be done before and after any definite exercise regimen.
- A person who wants to have an exercise programme after years of sedentary living should first have a pre-exercise physical examination with both cardiovascular and musculo-skeletal evaluation. Many cardiologists recommend graded treadmill exercises for persons with a history of cardiac disorder to know about the base data of physical work capacity and abnormal response to exercise. The result's of this testing provide guidelines for a safe and effective exercise programme.
- A person with a below average physical work capacity or a significant abnormal response to exercise should enter a supervised cardiac rehabilitations programme.
- A sedentary adult with normal capacity and exercise response should begin with an exercise programme slowly. Start with walking slowly and then over a period increase the pace and walk fast. When able to walk 2-3 km at a stretch without undue fatigue, can walk for 100 meters and jog for 50-100 meters thus gradually increasing the period of jogging over a period

time. Doing too much and too soon may result in injury and threat an enjoyable and healthful exercise programme.

- ❑ Low impact aerobic exercises such as swimming, cycling can strengthen and tone up muscles without over-straining.
- ❑ If not accustomed to, avoid activities that place undue stress or require sudden movement such as football, rowing, ballet, weight lifting or jogging till muscles are well trained. Get a personal assessment from a professional and follow an exercise regimen tailored to your needs.

Check List

- ❑ In bed sleep on your back with pillow under your knees or sleep on your side with legs bent. Choose a bed whose height makes it easy for you to get in and out. Do not sleep on stomach. Do not sleep on sofas or chairs.

Sitting

- ❑ Use an upright chair with arms, and back support. If possible have a chair with adjustable features.
- ❑ While sitting in chair support your back with a small cushion or a lumbar support.
- ❑ Keep your feet flat on the ground or on footrest.
- ❑ Get-up and stretch every 20-30 minutes.

Standing

- ❑ Stand tall with your stomach and buttocks tucked in.
- ❑ Avoid prolonged bending as when washing.

Walking

- ❑ Use comfortable low healed footwear.
- ❑ Walk erect and straight with arms relaxed and lightly swinging.

In Car

- ❑ Adjust your seat so that your arms are relaxed and bent at 90 degrees to the steering wheel.
- ❑ Support your lower back with a cushion.

At Work

- ❑ Avoid working in wrong posture, avoid bending your back.
- ❑ Work surface should be at a comfortable height.
- ❑ Choose to push or pull whenever possible, to lifting heavy unaccustomed weights.
- ❑ Lift only that much you are comfortable with. While lifting, bend your knees and avoid twisting. Keep your back straight and feet apart. Don't lift and twist simultaneously.
- ❑ Always lift and carry weight close to your body.
- ❑ Bend your knees rather than your back while putting a load down.
- ❑ Take breaks regularly and if possible take your break and lunch away from your workstation.
- ❑ Exercise while you sit to work and relax the muscles.
- ❑ Change your position throughout the day to avoid muscular strain.
- ❑ Change your feet position regularly and move your toes periodically.

Follow an exercise plan recommended by your medical professional. If possible, plan your day so that you perform varied tasks during the day.

4

Fitness is a Lifelong Process: Obesity in the Menopausal Zone

I. INTRODUCTION

Most of the women start expanding their waistline as they enter menopausal zone by crossing the magic figure of 40 years of age. However blaming the hormones alone for the obesity at this age; would be going too far. It is the faulty attitudes and lifestyles that are mainly responsible for the loss of figure due to protruding tummies and heavy hips. It is the intake of energy-dense foods and sedentary lifestyle that is responsible for the increase in deadly cargo; your own weight, and that gives the appearance of *bebeji early enough.* However, at the time of menopause women are additionally affected by the withdrawal of estrogens, which are protective to heart and also affect body metabolism. It leads to increased rates of all causes of mortality, viz. hypertension, diabetes mellitus and coronary artery disease. Overweight people are more likely to have high blood pressure and high blood cholesterol, major risk factors for heart disease and stroke. As people gain weight, their glucose tolerance declines putting overweight people at twice the risk for developing non-insulin-dependent diabetes mellitus (NIDDM/Type 2 diabetes). Diabetes is a major cause of early death, heart disease, kidney disease, stroke and blindness.

Several types of cancers are also associated with being overweight, including cancer of the uterus, gallbladder, cervix, ovary, breast and colon. Other conditions linked with obesity include sleep apnea, osteoarthritis, gout, gallbladder disease and infertility. Obesity-related conditions worsen as weight increases and often improve as the obesity is successfully treated. Weight gain around your waist (specifically in your abdominal area) is more of a health risk because it is more metabolically active than weight gained on your hips and thighs. Excess abdominal fat is associated with an increase in blood cholesterol and insulin resistance, which may result in diabetes. An "apple shaped" figure may also raise your risks for other life threatening illnesses, such as heart disease and stroke.

Weight loss can reverse most of the above complications and reduce the number and dosages of medications used. In order to accomplish this, lifestyle modifications are essential. The three parts of a successful weight-loss program are a proper diet, behavioural changes and physical activity. The prevention of obesity; the mother of several top killers should start during childhood. It is well known that a fat daughter will grow into a fat mother. Thus, obesity is unwelcome; mother or daughter. It is amusing to see a large number of fat looking middle-aged women regularly queuing up in front of pizza-huts along with plump children, instead of planning to take any exercise whatsoever.

2. OBESITY PREVALENCE

The prevalence of obesity in our times is steadily increasing. Majority of women from the so-called well-off section of society are overweight. Overweight individual is defined as one whose body mass index (BMI; the weight in kg divided by the square of height in meters) is above 25 kg/m. The definition of obesity requires a BMI of over 30 kg/m. It appears that more than one-third of well-off people in India have a BMI over 27.8 kg/m. Among the women in a study abroad among aged 50-59, 52% were overweight. The causes of this obesity can be divided into two major factors: genetic and environmental. The genetics accounts for a part of the risk of becoming obese. The environmental basis for the growing number of obese individuals is of great importance. Since we no longer need to chase wildlife or climb trees for procuring food, instead we just open the refrigerator door and start hogging, the results are obvious. The abundance of large food chains offering "super size deals" or "all you can eat", are in the competition for the consumers' money, larger portion sizes of high-energy foods are offered—and accepted with great perils to health. It is suggested that vegetables and grains should cover two-thirds of the plate. It is often recommended to eat plenty of fruits, vegetables and grains while limiting intake of red meat, alcohol, fat and salt. Several organizations advocate engagement in physical activity and avoidance of weight gain and cessation of smoking. The use of motorized vehicles, escalators and lifts has greatly decreased the amount of energy spent throughout the day. However, the number one enemy is the television set to which most women are glued throughout the day, which largely contributes to physical inactivity. Instead of watching T.V. riding a bicycle or jogging along with your children can be more healthful as well as joyful. Physical inactivity seems to play a major role in making you moribund. Menopause has been generally associated with lower energy expenditure and lower levels of physical activity leading to greater abdominal fat deposit. Estrogen is believed to protect the fertile female from cardiovascular diseases, including a better lipid profile, decreased coagulation and direct vascular effects. The use of HRT is believed to improve the plasma lipid profile, and is therefore expected to offer protection from the atherosclerotic process and coronary artery disease. Additionally, use of HRT has been shown to decrease the shift from gynoid (buttocks) to android (abdominal) fat deposits.

3. DIAGNOSIS

An excess of body fat results from an imbalance between energy intake and energy expenditure (i.e., consuming more calories than are needed). The reasons for this imbalance are unclear, and the relationship between energy intake/expenditure and body fat storage and distribution varies from person to person. Factors that promote obesity include: A genetic predisposition, Family history of obesity, Age, Behavioural factors (including a high-fat or high calorie diet and sedentary lifestyle), Biochemical differences (lower metabolic rate or decreased ability to oxidize fat).

3.1 Measuring Obesity

Assessment of your weight to determine if you are obese involves three key measurements—body mass index (BMI), waist circumference and consideration of risk factors for conditions associated with obesity. First you should determine your body mass index (BMI), which describes body weight relative to height and is strongly correlated with total body fat content in adults. A woman or man with a BMI between 25 and 29.9 is considered overweight; 30 or more is considered obese and 40 or greater is considered severely obese. Women in the highest obesity category have four times the risk of hypertension and/or high blood cholesterol than women of normal weight. Your doctor is more likely to conduct one or more of the following tests:

(a) Measuring Skin-fold Thickness

It measures subcutaneous fat, which lies just under the skin, at targeted areas such as the back of your upper arm, waist or thigh using calipers, an instrument that looks like tongs. Measurements of skin-fold thickness depend on the skill of the examiner and may vary widely when measured by different examiners.

(b) Bioelectrical Impedance

Using a handheld instrument called an impedance analyzer that transmits a non-invasive low frequency electrical current through electrodes placed on your hand and/or foot using a gel. Sophisticated software analyzes your body composition in seconds.

(c) Waist Circumference

It is strongly associated with abdominal fat, which is

an independent predictor of disease risk. Unlike fat around the thighs, which is more common in women and is more likely to serve as an energy reservoir, abdominal fat deposits are metabolically active: they deliver fatty acids directly into the bloodstream for immediate short-term energy. Higher proportions of this visceral fat are associated with higher risks of insulin resistance, diabetes, high blood pressure, heart disease and stroke.

3.2 Apple or Pear

How can you estimate your body fat distribution? Look at yourself in the mirror. If you are more apple-shaped than pear-shaped, you probably have visceral fat accumulation. Women with a waist circumference over 35 inches (and men over 40 inches) are at great risk. Your may do the following: Look at your personal weight history, Ask whether you have relatives with illnesses related to being overweight, such as Type 2 diabetes mellitus or heart disease, Discuss the methods you have used to lose weight in the past, Evaluate your risk for obesity-related health problems by measuring your blood pressure and doing blood tests

3.3 Let the Physician know

It is important that you tell your physician if you have any of the following as she assesses your condition:

- ❑ Pregnancy or breast feeding.
- ❑ History of gout or gallstones.
- ❑ History of drug or alcohol abuse.
- ❑ History of an eating disorder.
- ❑ History of depression or bipolar disorder.
- ❑ Use of monoamine oxidase (MAO) inhibitors or antidepressant medications.
- ❑ Migraine headaches requiring medication.
- ❑ Glaucoma.
- ❑ Diabetes.
- ❑ Heart disease or heart condition, such as an irregular heart beat.
- ❑ High blood pressure.
- ❑ Planning on surgery that requires general anesthesia.

You might also consult an endocrinologist. Endocrinologists are physicians who care for patients with complex hormonal disorders and metabolic conditions, including obesity, diabetes, thyroid disorders, metabolic bone disease, pituitary and adrenal conditions, and growth and gonadal disorders.

4. OBESITY-RELATED ILLNESSES

It is important to appreciate the average daily activities of obese women. Obese women exhibit more overall pain, less ability in physical functioning and lower self-esteem. The obese has difficulties in lifting and carrying heavy loads, climbing stairs, bending and vacuuming. The pain from being at a BMI of over 29 kg/m is found to be similar to that of having arthritis. This is the starting point for an otherwise "healthy" obese woman without any complications. The health problems associated with obesity are numerous, often hazardous, interfering with the quality of life and sometimes fatal. In plain words obesity maims and kills or, as has been said, "the obese dig their graves with their teeth." It has been estimated that lacks of annual deaths in India are attributed to being overweight and obese. It has been found that women with a BMI greater than 29 kg/m have four times the risk of death from cardiovascular disease when compared with those of a BMI less than 19 kg/m. The women with the highest waist-hip ratios have a high risk of death from coronary artery disease, compared to the leanest. Even a BMI within the recommended range may pose a threat. Women with BMIs of 23-24.9 kg/m already have an increased risk of 43% for heart attacks, when compared with fellow women with BMIs less than 21 kg/m. Regarding atherosclerosis-promoting illnesses, even a weight gain of a few kilograms may increase the risk of non-insulin dependant diabetes mellitus (NIDDM) two-fold, Gaining over 8 kg increased the risk almost three-fold, and women who gained over 20 kg had a relative risk of over 12 for developing diabetes. There seems to be a definite co-relation between abdominal fat and insulin resistance. The greater influx of free fatty acids from abdominal fat into the liver could act as a regulator of insulin levels, decreasing its breakdown and allowing for higher systemic levels. Eventually, insulin resistance develops. Hence, a diabeto-genic abdominal fat should be avoided. Also total and subcutaneous fats are not "safe" in terms of health hazards, and may promote the development of estrogen-related cancers. The risk for developing hypertension also grows with increasing body mass. Each of these two conditions is a "killer" on its own, but can combine to promote the development of atherosclerosis the basis for coronary artery disease and stroke. The presence of NIDDM greatly raises the risk for coronary events, stroke and all-cause-mortality, both independently and further in conjunction with hypertension, smoking or obesity. The relative risk for ischemic stroke among women with BMI of 27-28.9 kg/m is 75% higher when compared with the leanest. Women with higher BMIs have a greater prevalence of kidney stones. Gall bladder disease also occurs more in women with higher BMIs. For example, women with a BMI of 32 kg/m have 6 times the risk for developing gall stone disease when compared with the leanest. Osteoarthritis is another condition brought about by the increased weight. The difficulty with this illness is that the accompanying pain may prevent weight-bearing physical activity, which is needed for weight reduction. Pulmonary emboli (PE) were also found with increased incidence among the overweight and obese. Women with a BMI over 29 kg/m have three times the chance of suffering from PE. Of extreme importance is the relationship between obesity and malignancies. The incidence of breast cancer varies according to weight and weight gain. Even though a high BMI at the age of 18 carries a decreased risk of breast cancer (perhaps due to associated anovulation and lower endogenous estrogen levels), weight gain carried an elevated risk. Non-users of hormonal replacement therapy who gain over 20 kg in 16 years have twice the risk of breast cancer after menopause when compared to those with unchanged weight. Women who gain between 10-20 kg have a 60% higher risk. Unfortunately, overweight and obese women are less likely to be screened for breast and cervical cancers, even given their increased risk. This could possibly be due to a lower 'health awareness', which causes the increased weight and the screening negligence. Endometrial cancer is also found to be more prevalent among the obese. The explanation could be a higher level of estrogens originating from subcutaneous, non-visceral, fat tissue; meaning that reducing the amount of this tissue should also be targeted during weight loss. The incidence of colon adenomas, which are pre-cancerous lesions, is higher among women with higher BMIs. Women whose high BMI is due to central obesity have a higher risk than those with same BMI but less abdominal obesity. Adenocarcinoma of the esophagus and gastric cardia is also associated with increasing BMI in a dose-dependent manner and the effect is stronger in women than in men. Kidney cancer also has a greater prevalence among the obese. Additional relevant risk factors for this tumor are hypertension and smoking. Lung cancer is also found with increased frequency among the obese. Subjects with a BMI over 30 kg/m have twice the odds of developing lung cancer than the leanest. Despite this long list of complications, post-menopausal woman may find some advantages in obesity, especially regarding osteoporosis. The reasons for this could be either a direct effect of weight on weight-bearing bones, a hormonal effect from estrogen production in fat tissue which supports bone mass or a combination of the two. In a study of 8059 women aged over 65 years, the leanest had a risk of twice or more for fractures of the pelvis, hip and ribs.

5. WEIGHT LOSS REVERSES THE COMPLICATIONS OF OBESITY

Even a modest weight loss, that is 5-10 percent of initial weight, can lower or abolish the need for antihypertensive medications. In a study, women over 55 years of age who had lost over 10 kg over 16 years had a 15% less chance of developing hypertension. Insulin sensitivity also improves by reduction of abdominal fat, together with an improvement in blood lipid profile. Gallstone disease is less prevalent among the leaner, but obese individuals beginning weight loss can cause asymptomatic stones to become evident, so caution must be taken. Weight loss also eases the physical burden on the joints; thus the chance of developing osteoarthritis is less. For overweight women, every 2 units of BMI reduced yield a 60% reduction in the risk for symptomatic osteoarthritis.

5.1 Methods of Weight Reduction

Several methods are available for weight reduction: lifestyle modifications, medications or surgery. 'Magic diets' and special food additives are not important, as most have not been proved as beneficial over the long-term. The medications currently used for weight loss act to reduce energy intake, either by reducing appetite or inhibiting fat absorption. Drugs are modestly effective in reducing weight, by an average addition of 2-10 kg to a weight loss program. They are usually prescribed to those with BMIs over 27 kg/m, or with over 30% body fat for women. Patients with lower BMIs but with obesity-related conditions could also be treated with drugs. Currently, anti-obesity drugs are not recommended for routine use, and if initiated should be combined with the lifestyle changes.

5.2 Medicines or Surgery not the Choice of Intervention

It is doubtful whether drug treatment should be used for long-term management. Rather, medications should be compared to crutches for a person with a broken leg; temporary help until she can mange on her own, and probably for not more than 36 months. Gastric surgery is a very efficient method for weight reduction. It is currently reserved for patients with a BMI of over 40 kg/m who clearly understand the need for strict follow-up. Patients with a BMI over 35 kg/m may also be candidates for surgery if they have severe impairment in everyday living. Though effective, weight loss through surgery may not provide the additional benefits of lifestyle modification, such as proper food selection and engagement in exercise. The advantages of lifestyle modification are: it is simple, has no side effects, is possible to engage in over many years and puts weight reduction under the control of the patient. Hence, one can aim for a reasonable target weight, so osteoporosis may be avoided. Even a modest weight loss is beneficial. Additional benefits are the enhancement of mood and a better chance for cessation of smoking. The nutritional plan for weight loss, which is rich in grains, fruits and vegetables, may have additional effects such as decreased incidence of coronary artery disease, stroke or cancer. The combined lifestyle measures can offer greater protection from coronary heart disease, adding to the effects of weight loss. Overeating after surgery or cessation of drug use or exercise will eventually lead to a return to the initial weight.

6. LIFESTYLE MODIFICATION FOR TREATMENT OF OBESITY

The safest and most rewarding method of reducing excess weight is through a combination of three arms: proper diet, behavioural changes, adequate exercises and an attitude of fitness.

Diet

Dieting only is an effective way to lose weight, but not to maintain it very well. The parallel reduction of muscle mass might lower the metabolic rate and reduce energy expenditure, resulting in lower energy needs. Exercises can help to restore the amount of this energy-utilizing tissue. A minimal intake of 1200 kcal per day should be provided for women. It is probably advisable for subjects on a diet for longer than a couple of months to take a regular multivitamin supplement with extra calcium for women. Compliance to the nutritional program can be boosted by allowing at least one free day per week, when three "normal" meals may be consumed without any feelings of guilt.

Behavioural Changes

As obesity cannot be cured, but only managed, there is a need for life-long changes in certain habits. While transient reduction of weight can quite easily be accomplished, behaviour has a major role in the maintenance of the newly reduced body weight. The goal of changing everyday behaviour is, in fact, to reduce food intake and increase energy loss through exercises, thereby assisting the two other arms of lifestyle modification. Even though the need to combat obesity is lifelong, this may not be a lifelong struggle. Duration of weight maintenance is inversely related to effort involved. Another behavioural issue is smoking. It is not recommended to stop smoking along with decreasing food intake. Twenty-three percent of weight maintainers quit this habit, compared to only 13% of weight losers. Conversely, an increase in BMI elevated the chance of smoking cessation two-fold. In summary, the importance of behavioural changes is to assist in reducing food intake and increase daily energy output through activity.

7. PHYSICAL ACTIVITY IS THE BEST

Despite the numerous advantages to be described below, most of the women in menopausal zone do not report doing any regular physical activity. Even physicians do not promote fitness through active life and tend to recommend exercises as a form of secondary prevention. The 'at risk' population will therefore remain at risk. Regular exercises decrease mortality rates and this effect is also true for post-menopausal women as well. A low level of fitness is associated with increased mortality risk. In women, the moderately fit had a 55% reduction in mortality rates when compared with the least fit. In another study it appeared that obese but fit men were better-off than their lean and unfit counterparts. The unfit lean men had twice the chance of cardiovascular and all-cause mortality than the fit obese or lean men. Women over the age of 75, who are more active, may show a 75% reduction in mortality compared to the least active. This advocates mild to moderate activity even in this age group. One may have to continue an active lifestyle in order to enjoy its benefits. Still, one may also 'join the party' anytime and regain some protection, as compared to her/his sedentary friends. The concomitant reduction of traditional cardiovascular risk factors by exercises in women could also contribute to decreased morbidity and mortality. The more fit have a lower chance of smoking, having high blood pressure or having high cholesterol. Additionally, it may also prevent the accumulation of such fat during ageing and prevent weight gain. As central obesity is a contributor to insulin resistance and hypertension, reduction in these factors also follows. In both the obese and the non-obese, regular exercises reduces the risk for developing diabetes along the years. Regarding hypertension, physical fitness in women seemed to protect against development of hypertension. The blood lipid profile also improves with exercises. Stroke is another obesity-related but preventable complication. The suggested mechanism for stroke prevention is, therefore, slowing of the atherosclerotic process. Exercises can also combat additional obesity-related illnesses, e.g. risk for several types of cancers. Exercises have been known to Combat Gallbladder Disease and Osteoarthritis as well.

On average, the risk for cholecystectomy was 30% lower among the most active women when compared to their sedentary counterparts. Osteoarthritis can also be treated through a carefully planned exercise program. The type of exercise recommended for weight loss is of the aerobic type, such as walking, jogging, swimming, cycling and aerobic dancing. The older women seem to lose weight more easily than the younger. Women seem to need to work harder than men for the same weight loss but on the bright side, they will enjoy more hours of jogging in the outdoors. The rate of weight reduction should approximate 0.5 kg per week, by a combination of a reduced energy diet and exercises. As loss of 1 kg of body weight utilizes about 7000 kcal, the total energy deficit should therefore be about 500 kcal per day, resulting in a total of 3500 kcal per week. It should be stated that reduction of 500 kcal per day is much easier than increasing the expense of the same magnitude (for example, one hour of playing basketball). Minimal frequency of exercises is 3 times a week, while it is preferable to do so more often. The duration of exercise should be at least 30 minutes, which can be split into 2 or three bouts. Other measures include getting out of the elevator 3 floors below destination, parking farther away and looking after a dog. Since changing exercise behaviour is difficult, and it is no wonder that a large number of physicians still do not recommend moderate regular exercises for all adults, irrespective of weight. Losing as little as a five to 10 percent of body weight and maintaining that loss can significantly improve the health of obese patients by increasing glucose tolerance and lowering blood pressure and cholesterol levels. Therefore, if you are obese, you should seek medical help to lose weight as well as to maintain it. To be successful at achieving weight loss goals to improve your health, experts recommend losing weight at a rate of no more than one to two pounds per week, and then maintaining that loss for six months before losing more. Maintaining weight loss can be more difficult than losing the weight to begin with. The good news is that by burning-off more calories than you're taking in will cause you to lose weight. The safest way to lose weight is to eat a nutritionally complete diet that is moderate in calories and fat and add exercise to your daily routine.

8. CHANGING YOUR DIET

As a rule of thumb, if you take in about 250 calories per day less than is needed to maintain your current weight, combined with an exercise regime that burns an additional 250 calories a day, you will lose about a pound per week. Multiply your current weight by 10. For example, a woman who weighs 100 pounds requires 1,000 calories per day to maintain bodily functions like breathing and digestion. You need additional calories—about 30 percent to 50 percent more if you are moderately active—to provide energy for daily activities like walking, vacuuming, even sitting at the computer. To satisfy basic nutritional needs, eat a variety of foods every day by choosing from each of the five food groups—milk, meat, fruit, vegetable and grains. While you should try to cut back on fats and sugars, all foods and beverages can be consumed in moderation. Balanced food plans encourage making wise choices about everyday food—choices you can make to stay at your proper weight for life. Many popular diet plans—the high protein/low carbohydrate diet, for example—don't include balanced choices. While women can lose weight on these diets, they can be dangerously deficient in certain required nutrients or food groups and dangerously high in others. Most successful weight-loss plans call for a reduction in both calories and fat, although fat is probably not a critical component in obesity. Instead, overall calories and lack of physical activity, coupled with a sedentary lifestyle, are. Dietary guidelines recommend women moderate their fat consumption to 25 or less of your total calorie intake, with saturated fats accounting for only about 10 percent of intake and comprised of equal amounts of monounsaturated fat and polyunsaturated fats—that is, more vegetable-source fats. Also, reduce cholesterol intake to about 300 mg per day. Increase your consumption of fruits, vegetables and whole grains.

8.1 Add Exercise to the Dieting Program

Exercise on the other hand, not only burns calories, it also tempers the appetite. Exercise boosts metabolism, which dieting can impair, improves sleep and provides psychological benefits, such as an increased feeling of control and self-esteem, as well as stress reduction. If you are over 40, have been inactive for some time, suffer from shortness of breath or weakness that interferes with daily activities, or suffer from a chronic condition, you should consult a physician before you begin your effort to increase your physical activity. Be sure to notify your physician about any chest pain, faintness or dizziness, bone or joint pain and any medications you may be taking. The best kinds of exercises for burning calories are aerobic activities, which involve using the large muscles of your body in a rhythmic, continuous activity. Aerobics not only help to reduce body fat but also improve cardiovascular conditioning. While you should set-up a detailed exercise plan based on your individual health status, they recommend healthy women do some sort of moderate-to-vigorous aerobic exercise on most or all days of the week for 30 to 45 minutes. These minutes can be accumulated—15 minutes of an aerobics in the morning and 15 minutes of brisk walking in the evening, for example. However, a single sustained exercise session may be more effective in helping you to lose weight. If you have been inactive, you need to work up slowly so that you don't get injured or overly fatigued and then discouraged. Start with five or 10 minutes—or whatever you're comfortable with—every other day, and add one minute every other session. Low—to moderate-intensity aerobic exercise, like housework, gardening and walking with the dog, provide a great deal of general health benefits, but for weight loss, you need to up the ante and exercise at a higher intensity with vigorous activities like brisk walking or jogging, singles tennis/racket sports, aerobics classes, ice or roller skating, swimming or cycling.

8.2 Measure Heart Rate

Because the goal of aerobic exercise is to work your heart muscle, your exercise needs to increase your heart rate. One-way to determine if you are exercising intensely enough is to measure your heart rate. After warming up and then sustaining an aerobic activity for about five minutes, take your pulse by placing two fingers on the carotid artery on the side of your neck, just under your jaw line and about one to two inches in front of your ear. Count the beats for 10 seconds. Your heart rate should be about 70 percent to 85 percent of its maximum, which is your age subtracted from 220. The following chart illustrates recommended 10-second heart rate counts; the number of beats you count should fall between the two numbers listed beside your age.

Age	*70 % of maximum*	*85 % of maximum*
20	23	28
30	22	27
40	21	26
50	20	24
60	18	23

If you are out of shape or older than 60, you should aim for an intensity at 50 to 70 percent of your maximum heart rate. To determine what your heart rate should be during exercise, subtract your age from 220; divide that number by six for a 10-second heart rate count, then multiply that number by 0.6 for the lower end of the range and 0.73 for the higher end. For example, if you're 70:

- ❑ 220 – 70 = 150 (this would be your maximum heart rate for one minute).
- ❑ 150 x 6 = 25 (this would be your maximum heart rate for 10 seconds).
- ❑ 25 x 0.60 = 15 (this would be 60 percent of your maximum, or the lower end of where your 10-second heart rate should be when you're exercising).
- ❑ 25 x 0.73 = 18 (this would be 73 percent of your maximum, or the higher end of where your 10-second heart rate should be when you're exercising).

An easier way to judge intensity is the "talk test." You shouldn't be exercising so hard that you can't talk with a friend or recite a poem. If you can't talk without gasping for breath, slow down. On the other hand, if your exercise is easy enough that you can sing a song out loud, you probably need to increase your intensity.

8.3 Strength Training may Help as Well

Another type of exercise is strength training—which includes weight lifting and isometrics, or using your own body weight as resistance such as in push ups—not only improves muscular strength and endurance, it also raises metabolism, causing you to burn more calories. Make sure you take a few minutes to stretch and warm up before doing any kind of exercise. It's best to incorporate a combination of both types of exercise into your lifestyle—aerobics to burn fat and strength training to build muscle—because neither type is as effective alone. At the same time, you need to reduce the amount of television you watch, since TV watching is independently associated with obesity.

9. MEDICATIONS FOR TREATING OBESITY

Weight-loss medications may be recommended for patients who are at increased medical risk because of their obesity. Most research-based and professional associations recommend lifestyle therapy for at least six months before embarking on a weight-loss plan using physician-prescribed drug therapy. Currently, available prescription medications include:

- ❑ Phentermine (Adipex, Fastin, Ionamin, Oby-trim),
- ❑ Diethylpropion (Tenuate, Tenuate dospan, Tepanil),
- ❑ Mazindol (Sanorex, Mazanor),
- ❑ Phendimetrazine (Adipost, Bontril, Plegine, Prelu-2, X-Trozine),
- ❑ Benzphetamine (Didrex),
- ❑ Sibutramine (Meridia), and
- ❑ Orlistat (Xenical).

Most of these appetite-suppressants have been approved for short-term use, meaning a few weeks or months. Most of these drugs decrease appetite by affecting levels of the brain neurotransmitters catecholamine, serotonin and/or noradrenaline — brain chemicals that affect mood and appetite. In general, these medications are modestly effective. If you are, may be or could become pregnant or are nursing, be sure to tell your healthcare professional. You also will need to tell your doctor about any existing medical problems before taking these medications, especially thyroid problems, anxiety disorders, epilepsy or other seizure disorders, diabetes, heart disease, high blood pressure, arteriosclerosis, or glaucoma. Side effects of anti-obesity drugs can range from mild to serious.

9.1 Surgery

For clinically severe obesity, surgery may be an element of treatment. Surgery is an option for carefully selected patients under the care of a physician who:

(a) Have tried other methods of weight loss (changes in eating, behaviour, increased physical activity and/or drug therapy) and are still severely obese.

(b) Are unable to physically perform routine daily activities (work-related and family functions) and have a seriously impaired quality of life due to the severity of obesity.

(c) Understand the procedure, risks of surgery and effects after surgery.

(d) Are motivated to make a lifelong behavioural commitment that includes well-balanced eating and physical activity needed to achieve—and maintain—desired results.

There are two types of obesity surgery—restrictive and combined with malabsorptive. Restrictive surgery—also called a gastric bypass—uses surgically placed bands or staples to decrease the size of your stomach, creating a restriction in the amount of food you can eat. Possible complications include leaking of stomach juices into the abdomen, injury to the spleen, erosion of the band, breakdown of the staple line and the sectioned portion stretching from overeating. Infection or death has been reported in less than one percent of patients. After surgery, you have to learn to eat smaller amounts of food at one time, to chew food well and to eat slowly; if you don't adjust your eating habits, your weight loss will be inhibited. In addition, especially in the first three months after surgery, you must be sure to eat the proper amounts of protein, calories, minerals and vitamins. Eighty percent of restrictive surgery patients lose some weight; 30 percent reach normal weight. Equally important, the operation appears to resolve a variety of serious weight-related health problems. Diabetes, which is common in obese people and which can lead to blindness, nerve degeneration and death, is often much improved or even cured by the weight loss that occurs after a gastric bypass. Combined restrictive and malabsorptive surgery is a combination of restrictive surgery as described above with bypass or malabsorptive surgery, in which the stomach is connected to the small intestine, bypassing the duodenum, which is the beginning portion of the small intestine. The longer the segment of small intestine bypassed, the greater the malabsorption component—that is, the fewer the calories absorbed from the food you eat—and the greater the weight loss.

9.2 Surgery Involves Risks

There is a risk from this procedure for nutritional deficiencies including malabsorption of vitamin B12, leading to anemia and iron deficiency. The reduction in vitamin D and calcium absorption can cause osteoporosis and other bone disease. Other complications are similar to those of restrictive surgery and are due to creating the stomach pouch. After surgery, lifelong use of nutritional supplements such as multivitamins, vitamin B12, vitamin D and calcium is necessary, as is nutritional counseling. The "dumping syndrome" in which food moves too quickly through the small intestine can cause nausea, weakness, sweating, faintness and sometimes diarrhea after eating. There can also be an inability to eat sweets without severe weakness and sweating. Dairy intolerance, constipation, headache, hair loss and depression are other possible side effects.

9.3 Include Helpful Behavioural Strategies

(i) *Set the Right Goals*: your goals should focus on specific dietary and exercise changes, such as "I will eat five servings of fruits and vegetables every day this week," or "I will work up to being able to walk briskly for 30 minutes at a time," rather than just on weight loss.

(ii) *Reward success*: To encourage yourself to attain your goals, reward yourself for successes. An effective reward is something that is desirable and timely.

(iii) *Keep a food and exercise daily*: Many behavioural psychologists believe it's necessary to track your daily food consumption to achieve long-term weight loss.

(iv) *Monitor your weight sensibly*: Keep track of your weight, but don't weigh too often. One day's diet and exercise patterns won't have a measurable effect on the scale the next day, and your body's water weight can change from day-to-day, which may frustrate you and derail your efforts.

(v) Find ways other than food to respond to stress and other situations in your life.

(vi) *Change the way you go about eating*: There are a variety of tricks, from using a smaller plate to eating more slowly, that can help you eat less.

10. FAQ ON OBESITY

Q. What is Obesity?

To most people, the term "obesity" means to be very overweight. Health professionals define "overweight" as an excess amount of body weight that includes muscle, bone, fat, and water. "Obesity" specifically refers to an excess amount of body fat. Some people, such as body-builders or other athletes with a lot of muscle, can be overweight without being obese.

Q. How is Obesity Measured?

Everyone needs a certain amount of body fat for stored energy, heat insulation, shock absorption, and other functions. As a rule, women have more body fat than men. Most health care providers agree that men with more than 25 percent body fat and women with more than 30 percent body fat are obese. Measuring the exact amount of a person's body fat is not easy. The most accurate measures are to weigh a person underwater or to use an X-ray test called Dual Energy X-ray Absorptiometry (DEXA). These methods are not practical. There are simpler methods to estimate body fat. One is to measure the thickness of the layer of fat just under the skin in several parts of the body. Another involves sending a harmless amount of electricity through a person's body. Both methods are used at health clubs and commercial weight loss programs. Results from these methods, however, can be inaccurate if done by an inexperienced person or on someone with severe obesity. Weight-for-height tables, which have been used for decades, usually have a range of acceptable weights for a person of a given height. One problem with these tables is that there are many versions, all with different weight ranges. In recent years, body mass index (BMI) has become the medical standard used to measure overweight and obesity.

Q. What is Body Mass Index?

BMI uses a mathematical formula based on a person's height and weight. BMI equals weight in kilograms divided by height in meters squared (BMI = kg/m^2). Although the BMI ranges shown in the graph are not exact ranges of healthy and unhealthy weight, they are useful guidelines. A BMI of 25 to 29.9 indicates a person is overweight. A person with a BMI of 30 or higher is considered obese. Like the weight-to-height table, BMI does not show the difference between excess fat and muscle. BMI, however, is closely associated with measures of body fat. It also predicts the development of health problems related to excess weight. For these reasons, BMI is widely used by health care providers.

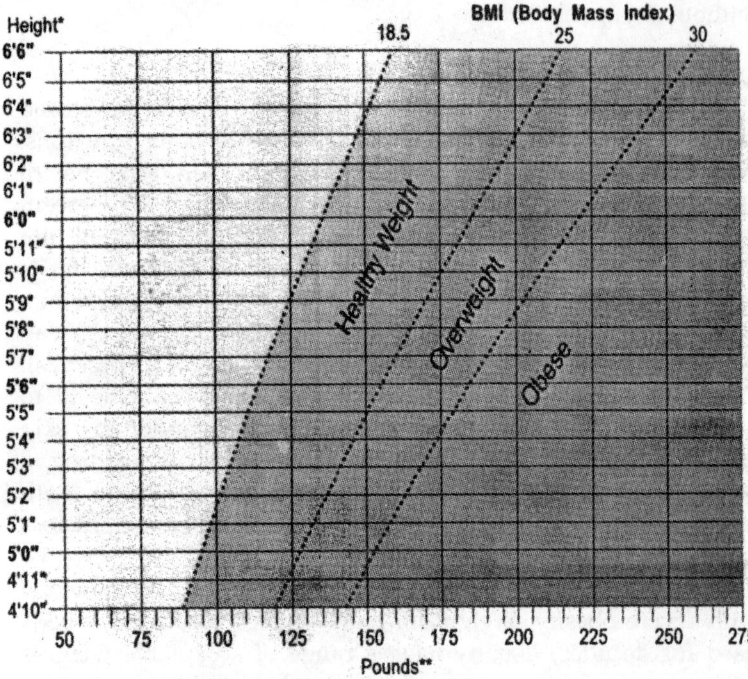

Find your weight on the bottom of the graph. Go straight up from that point until you come to the line that matches your height. Then look to find your weight group.

Q. What is "Pears" vs. "Apples"?

Health care providers are concerned not only with how much fat a person has, but also where the fat is located on the body. Women typically collect fat in their hips and buttocks, giving them a "pear" shape. Men usually build-up fat around their bellies, giving them more of an "apple" shape. Of course, some men are pear-shaped and some women become apple-shaped, especially after menopause. If you carry fat mainly around your waist, you are more likely to develop obesity-related health problems. Women with a waist measurement of more than 35 inches or men with a waist measurement of more than 40 inches have a higher health risk because of their fat distribution.

Q. What are the Causes of Obesity?

In scientific terms, obesity occurs when a person consumes more calories than he or she burns. What causes this imbalance between calories in and calories out may differ from one person to another. Genetic, environmental, psychological, and other factors may all play a part.

Q. What are the Genetic Factors in Obesity?

Obesity tends to run in families, suggesting a genetic cause. Yet families also share diet and lifestyle habits that may contribute to obesity. Separating these from genetic factors is often difficult. Even so, science shows that heredity is linked to obesity. In one study, adults who were adopted as children were found to have weights closer to their biological parents than to their adoptive parents. In this case, the person's genetic make-up had more influence on the development of obesity than the environment in the adoptive family home.

Q. What are Environmental Factors in Obesity?

While Genes do have influence people, environment also strongly influences obesity. This includes lifestyle behaviours such as what a person eats and his or her level of physical activity. Rich people in India tend to eat high-fat foods, and put taste and convenience ahead of nutrition. Also, most of them do not get enough physical activity. Although you cannot change your genetic make-up, you can change your eating habits and levels of activity. Try these techniques that have helped some people lose weight and keep it off:

- ❑ Learn how to choose more nutritious meals that are lower in fat.
- ❑ Learn to recognize and control environmental cues (like inviting smells) that make you want to eat when you're not hungry.
- ❑ Become more physically active.
- ❑ Keep records of your food intake and physical activity.

Q. What is the Role of Psychological Factors?

Psychological factors may also influence eating habits. Many people eat in response to negative emotions such as boredom, sadness, or anger. Most overweight people have no more psychological problems than people of average weight. Still, up to 10 percent of people who are mildly obese and try to lose weight on their own or through commercial weight loss programs have binge eating disorder. This disorder is even more common in people who are severely obese. During a binge-eating episode, people eat large amounts of food and feel that they cannot control how much they are eating. Those with the most severe eating problems are also likely to have symptoms of depression and low self-esteem. These people may have more difficulty losing weight and keeping it off. If you are upset by binge eating behaviour and think you might have binge eating disorder, seek help from a health professional such as a psychiatrist, psychologist, or clinical social worker.

Q. What are the other Causes of Obesity?

Some illnesses can lead to obesity or a tendency to gain weight. These include hypothyroidism, Cushing's syndrome, depression, and certain neurological problems that can lead to overeating. Also, drugs such as steroids and some anti-depressants may cause weight gain. A doctor can tell whether there are underlying medical conditions that are causing weight gain or making weight loss difficult.

Q. What are the Consequences of Obesity?

Obesity is more than a cosmetic problem; it is a health hazard. Many deaths each year are related to obesity. Several serious medical conditions have been linked to obesity, including type 2 diabetes, heart disease, high blood pressure, and stroke. Obesity is also linked to higher rates of certain types of cancer. Obese men are more likely than non-obese men to die from cancer of the colon, rectum, or prostate. Obese women are more likely than non-obese women to die from cancer of the gallbladder, breast, uterus, cervix, or ovaries.

Other diseases and health problems linked to obesity include:

- Gallbladder disease and gallstones.
- Liver disease.
- Osteoarthritis, a disease in which the joints deteriorate. This is possibly the result of excess weight on the joints.
- Gout, another disease affecting the joints.
- Pulmonary (breathing) problems, including sleep apnea in which a person can stop breathing for a short time during sleep.
- Reproductive problems in women, including menstrual irregularities and infertility.

Q. What are the Psychological and Social Effects?

Emotional suffering may be one of the most painful parts of obesity. The society emphasizes physical appearance and often equates attractiveness with slimness, especially for women. Such messages make overweight people feel unattractive. Many people think that obese individuals are gluttonous, lazy, or both, even though this is not true. As a result, obese people often face prejudice or discrimination in the job market, at school, and in social situations. Feelings of rejection, shame, or depression are common.

Q. Who should lose weight?

Doctors generally agree that people who have a BMI of 30 or more can improve their health through weight loss. This is especially true for people who are severely obese. Preventing additional weight gain is recommended if you have a BMI between 25 and 29.9, unless you have other risk factors. Obesity experts recommend you try to lose weight if you have two or more of the following:

- *Family history of certain chronic diseases*: If you have close relatives who have had heart disease or diabetes, you are more likely to develop these problems if you are obese.
- *Pre-existing medical conditions*: High blood pressure, high cholesterol levels, or high blood sugar levels are all warning signs of some obesity-associated diseases.
- *"Apple" shape*: If your weight is concentrated around your waist, you may have a higher risk of heart disease, diabetes, or cancer than people of the same weight who have a "pear" shape.

Fortunately, a weight loss of 5 to 10 percent can do much to improve health by lowering blood pressure and cholesterol levels and also preventing diabetes.

Q. How is Obesity Treated?

The method of treatment depends on your level of obesity, overall health condition, and motivation to lose weight. Treatment may include a combination of diet, exercise, behaviour modification, and rarely weight-loss drugs. In some cases of severe obesity, gastrointestinal surgery may be recommended. Remember, weight control is a life-long effort.

Q. What's the difference between being obese and being overweight?

In both overweight and obese people, the defining characteristic is excess body fat. The difference is a matter of degree. Overweight people usually have a body mass index (BMI), or ratio of weight to height, of 25 to 29.9. Obesity is usually defined as a BMI of 30 or more. Another measure of obesity is having more than 30 percent body fat. While overweight people have a higher incidence of certain diseases and conditions than normal weight individuals, as people gain weight, they become even more prone to these often life-threatening problems.

Q. According to the charts, I'm categorized as obese, but I don't look fat, and I exercise at least five times a week, doing both aerobic exercises and weight training. What's going on?

Chances are you are one of the individuals who don't fit neatly into the BMI or height/weight charts because you have a significant amount of muscle, which weighs more than fat and makes your weight seem above the normal limits. What's really more important to consider is your body composition—your proportion of fat to muscle. As an avid exerciser and weight lifter, it's doubtful your body fat is greater than 30 percent.

Q. At 100 kg, I have more than 30 kgs to lose. I feel like I'll never achieve that. Should I just give up?

No. Losing as little as five to 10 percent of your body weight—can significantly improve your health.

Q. I realize I need to lose weight; how should I get started?

The safest way to lose weight is, in most cases, to eat a nutritionally complete diet that cuts about 250 calories a day from the number of calories your body requires to maintain its present weight, plus add an exercise regime that burns an additional 250 calories a day. If you do this, you will lose about a pound per week.

Q. Do I have to exercise to lose weight?

No, you don't have to. But not only will exercise make the weight come-off more quickly and easily, it will make your weight loss much easier to maintain. If you do lose the weight without exercising, you will still be unfit, which in itself is a health hazard.

Q. I've heard some nightmare stories about stomach stapling and other obesity-related surgical procedures. Are they safe?

For severe obesity, restrictive surgery (stomach stapling) and combined restrictive and malabsorptive surgery (in which the duodenum is bypassed) are safer than remaining severely obese consistent follow-up and patient compliance with post-surgical treatment is crucial to the success of these surgeries. These surgical procedures are used only in patients who have been unsuccessful at losing weight in other ways.

Q. How many people in India exercise?

In India most of the people, esp. from the prosperous background do not exercise or perform any physical activity at all. Even 60 percent of Americans don't meet basic activity level recommendations and 25 percent are completely sedentary.

Q. What is the importance of waist line?

If a woman's waist circumference is more than 35 inches, she is considered to have a high amount of visceral fat, which is the type of fat that surrounds the internal organs. This type of fat is associated with higher risk of certain diseases and conditions like diabetes and heart disease.

Q. Can children be overweight or obese?

Yes. Today, there are nearly twice as many overweight children and almost three times as many overweight adolescents as there were in 1980. Obesity is not acceptable even in children.

Q. Why are so many people overweight or obese today?

Behavioural and environmental factors are the main contributors to overweight and obesity and provide the greatest opportunities for prevention and treatment.

Q. How does overweight and obesity affect your health?

If you are overweight, you are more likely to develop health problems; such as, heart disease, stroke, diabetes, cancer (such as colon cancer, endometrial cancer, and post-menopausal breast cancer), gallbladder disease, sleep apnea (interrupted breathing during sleep), osteoarthritis (wearing away of the joints). The more overweight you are, the more likely you are to have health problems. Weight loss and regular exercise can help improve the harmful effects of being overweight. Studies show if you are overweight or obese, losing 5-10% of your body weight can improve your health.

Q. What can be done about this major public health problem?

It is essential to work together to prevent and reduce obesity through Communication—by educating, motivating, and empowering decision-makers at all levels to create healthier communities.

Q. What are the costs associated with overweight and obesity?

While Indian costs are not known, in the year 2000, the cost of obesity in the United States was more than $117 billion. Poor nutrition and physical inactivity account for some 300,000 premature deaths in the United States each year.

5

Essentials to Fitness: Prevention of Diseases and their Early Detection

HARSH MOHAN* AND ANNU NANDA**

Most doctors are attracted to medicine because they look forward to curing a disease. However, most patients would prefer never to contract a disease in the first place or, if they must contract an illness, they prefer that it be caught early and treated before it causes them any harm. In order to achieve this, many procedures are sometimes performed on patients without specific complaints, to identify risk factors or find disease early in its course, so that by intervening, patients can remain well. Such activity is referred to as the periodic health examination.

LEVELS OF PREVENTION

The dictionary defines prevention as "the act of keeping from happening." Depending on when the clinical efforts are made, three types of prevention are usually possible.

* MD, MNAMS, FICPath, UICC, Professor & Head, Department of Pathology, Government Medical College, Chandigarh.

** MD, Senior Resident, Government Medical College, Chandigarh.

Primary Prevention

Primary prevention keeps disease from occurring at all by removing risk factors. Immunization for many communicable diseases are examples of this kind of prevention, as is helping people to stop smoking.

Secondary Prevention

Secondary prevention detects disease early when it is still asymptomatic and when early treatment can stop the disease from progressing; Pap smears and other tests for occult malignancies are main examples. The role of a pathologist is mainly in this kind of prevention in helping in early diagnosis of the disease.

Tertiary Prevention

Tertiary prevention refers to those clinical activities that prevent further deterioration, for example, beta-blocking agents to reduce the risk of death in patients who have recovered from myocardial infarction.

Primary prevention is usually accomplished outside the health care system. In physicians' practice most effort is spent on tertiary prevention, less on secondary prevention and least on primary prevention.

PREVENTION

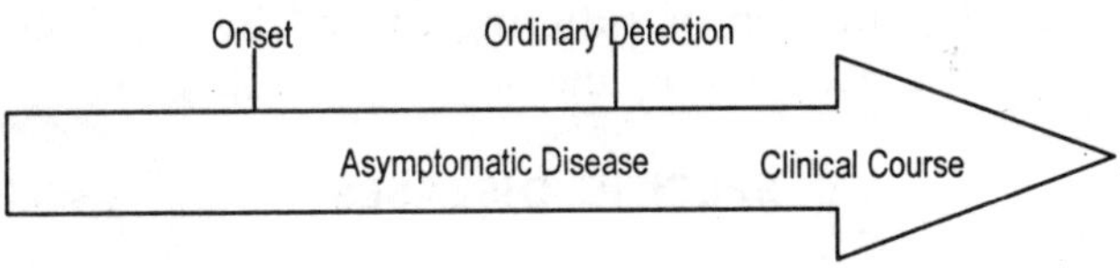

Primary	*Secondary*	*Tertiary*
Remove risk factors	Early detection and treatment	Reduce complications

SCREENING

One major activity in the prevention armamentarium is screening. The purpose of screening is either to detect individuals with risk factors that predispose to disease development in which case specific preventive interventions would be involved or to identify persons with early or asymptomatic (latent) disease that can be effectively treated leading to a better health outcome.

Screening has been defined as the presumptive identification of an unrecognized disease or defect by the application of tests, examinations or other procedures, which can be applied rapidly. Screening tests sort out apparently well persons who have a disease from those who probably do not. A screening test is not intended to be diagnostic. It helps in the prevention of a disease to a fatal outcome by means of early detection followed by definitive treatment. Screening is one component of early detection, which in return is one aspect of secondary prevention.

Which Disease to be Screened?

While considering which screening tests to be performed routinely on asymptomatic patients, a decision must first be made as to which medical problem or disease should be sought. Three criteria are important when deciding which medical condition should be sought during screening:

1. The effectiveness of the ensuing treatment if the condition is found.
2. The burden of suffering caused by the condition.
3. The accuracy of the screening test.

SPECIFIC DISEASES

Cancer

Neoplasms are diseases characterized by abnormal proliferation of cells. If the proliferating cells do not invade surrounding tissues, the resultant tumor is benign; if they do, it is malignant. The term 'cancer' includes all malignant tumors arising in body tissues. In any case early diagnosis and treatment prolong survival in most cases of cancer. It ought to be emphasized that most cancers are preventable.

In India, cancers are the third leading cause of death. There are 1.5-2 million cancer patients at any point of time. The incidence is estimated to be 70-80/100,000 per year. The commonest cancer in India in men is oropharyngeal cancer and in women cancer of cervix. Data from 6 metropolitan and one rural cancer registry in India show that the five most common cancers in India in men are cancer lung (10.6%), pharynx (9.1%), esophagus (6.7%), tongue (6.6%) and stomach (5.7%), while in women cancer cervix (23.5%), breast (19.3%), ovary (5.5%), esophagus (4.4%) and mouth (3.9%) are the most common sites.

Lung Cancer

Lung cancer is leading cause of cancer death worldwide. It accounts for 6.8% of all malignancies in India. It is a tragedy that the major cause has been known for a long time and is avoidable, i.e. smoking. There is a relatively long period between exposure and disease. This latency period thereby presents an opportunity to prevent the disease. Lung cancer is often diagnosed in a relatively late stage. Efforts at primary prevention (i.e., avoidance of risk factors) and secondary prevention (screening for early diagnosis) are therefore crucial to reduce the mortality due to lung cancer.

Risk Factors

Smoking

91% of lung cancer in men and 77% in women are attributable to cigarette smoking.

Occupational Exposure

Radon, asbestos, arsenic, chromium, polycyclic aromatic compounds, nickel, vinyl chloride have been recognized as risk factors.

Others

Chronic obstructive ling disease, foods high in fats, animal protein or cured meats. On the other hand, high intake of fruits and vegetables has a protective effect. (See Appendix I, 'Guidelines for the Management of chronic obstructive disease' for further details on this common problem)

Screening

The standard method for screening for lung cancer is:

1. Chest radiography.
2. Sputum cytology.

Studies have shown that screening for lung cancer in the general population despite increasing the detection does not improve the death rates. Screening is, however, worthwhile in individual patients documented to be at high risk.

Future Directions

In view of the inability of screening for early lung cancer to reduce mortality rate, attention has shifted to detecting early precursor lesions rather than looking for early lung cancer. Methods are being developed for identifying patients with pre-clinical disease and include a variety of methods for analyzing shed bronchial cells, fluorescence imaging to identify dysplastic lesions and cell analyzers for biomarkers.

Breast Cancer

The incidence of breast cancer is increasing; however, the mortality rate has remained about the same, perhaps reflecting earlier detection and improved management.

The following list enumeratcs some of the known risk factors. Patients are at a high risk of developing breast cancer if relative risk is greater than 4.0 (i.e., the chance of getting cancer breast is four times higher than in the general population). A modified relative risk factor is between 2.0-4.0 and low risk is considered to be 1.7-1.9.

Breast Cancer Risk Factors

High (relative risk >4)

- ❑ Age>65.
- ❑ Prior invasive or *in situ* carcinoma.

- Family history of 2 or more relatives with pre-menopausal and/or bilateral breast cancer.
- A typical hyperplasia on prior breast biopsy.
- Having been born in North America or Northern Europe.

Moderate (relative risk 2-4)

- Family history of first degree relative with breast cancer.
- Obesity.
- Age at first full term pregnancy of greater than 30 years.
- Nulliparity.
- History of prior ovarian or endometrian cancer.
- Prior radiation to the thorax.
- Mammographic pattern of dysplasia and prominent ductal tissue.

Low (relative risk 1-2)

- Alcohol consumption.
- Early menarche.
- Late menopause.

Breast Examination

It is recommended that a breast physical examination be done by a physician every 3 years between the ages of 20 and 40 years and annually thereafter. This is the most powerful tool in detecting early breast cancer. The best time to examine is one week after menstruation.

Breast Self-examination

Any abnormality found in the breast or axilla should be reported to the physician immediately. However, it is important to realize that 80% of lumps detected are actually benign.

Mammography

Breast cancer is one of the four malignancies for which the value of screening has been demonstrated in prospective randomized trials. Although cost-effectiveness estimates of breast cancer screening vary widely, the estimates available suggest that breast cancer screening is a cost effective public health strategy.

Cancer Cervix

The world-wide incidence of cervical cancer is second to breast cancer, but is the most common cancer in females in developing countries.

Risk factors

Socio-economic status is inversely related to the incidence of cervical carcinoma. The most compelling risk factors for carcinoma of the cervix is that it is a sexually transmitted disease due to an infectious agent. There is evidence that HPV (Human papilla virus) is etiologically related to cervical cancer.

Screening

Pap smear is an evaluation of cells from the cervical region by a cytologist/pathologist. Screening with pap smears has been shown to identify early lesions and thus decrease the incidence of invasive cancer and mortality due to cancer cervix. All the females should have a Pap test at the beginning of sexual activity, every 3 years thereafter and annually after 40 years of age. Pap smears have a false negative rate of 20-30% for a single smear in routine practice. The false negative rate will depend upon the ability of the individual taking the smear, the location and grade of the lesion, the accuracy of interpretation and the age of the patient.

Head and Neck Cancer

Oral cancer especially of the buccal mucosa is particularly common in South India and in states of U.P. and Bihar. It is estimated that 50,000 new cases occur annually in India. Oral cancer accounts for 28% of the total cancers in India and constitutes about 10% of all head and neck cancers.

The occurrence of oropharyngeal malignancy is strongly associated with the habit of chewing betel leaf, areca nut, and tobacco, as also with smoking. Certain paan masalas, whose use has markedly reduced during last few years, are also carcinogenic.

Prevention

- ❑ Oral cancers are amenable to primary prevention by eliminating the habit of tobacco chewing.
- ❑ Oral cancers are easily accessible for inspection allowing early detection. If detected early with the help of biopsy (microscopic examination by the pathologist) of the affected area, they can be treated or cured.

Infections

The incidence of infectious diseases has reduced considerably in the last hundred years due to better understanding of these conditions and application of effective methods of prevention and control. The extreme importance and potential effectiveness of preventive strategies to the population as a whole, rather than just the individual, seem to have caught the imagination of those at the forefront of medical research and practice. Some infections by virtue of their unique cause and effect nature are particularly susceptible to preventive strategies. This portion serves to highlight the important aspects of infections alterable by preventive measures.

I. Bacterial Diseases

Tuberculosis

This disease primarily affects lungs and can also affect intestines, meanings, bones and joints, lymph nodes, skin and other tissue of the body. India accounts for nearly one third of the global burden of tuberculosis. Every year approximately 2.2 million persons develop tuberculosis and about 5 lakh people die of tuberculosis every year.

Source of Infection

The reservoir is almost always a case of pulmonary

tuberculosis with positive sputum. Bacilli from lungs and bronchi of open cases come out in the form of droplets on coughing, sneezing, laughing and talking. Small droplets are inhaled directly. Unboiled milk or uncooked meat of diseased cattle may on ingestion rarely initiate intestinal tuberculosis.

Signs and Symptoms

Common symptoms are low-grade fever, especially in the evening, night sweats, loss of weight, and increase in ESR. There are three easily identifiable symptoms associated with tuberculosis:

1. Cough for > 21 days.
2. Chest pain for > 15 days.
3. Absence of expectoration.

Diagnosis

Direct examination of sputum

Direct microscopy of sputum is reliable, cheap and easy. Examination of two consecutive samples is sufficient to detect tuberculosis in large number of infectious cases.

AFB culture

It is difficult, lengthy (takes approx. 6 weeks) and expensive and is recommended only for patient with chest symptoms whose sputum smear is negative.

Chest X-ray

Field diagnostic surveys

Field diagnostic surveys are based on—

- Tuberculin test.
- Sputum examination.

Control and Prevention

Mantoux test

This test consists of introducing tuberculin, a protein of tubercle bacillus, into the skin and observing whether an allergic reaction develops or not. A positive reaction to the test is generally accepted as evidence of past or present tubercular infection.

Sputum Examination

Sputum culture

Leprosy

Leprosy is a chronic infectious disease affecting mainly the skin and peripheral nerves. It may also affects muscle, eyes, bones, testes and intestinal organs. The disease manifests itself in two polar forms: namely, lepromatous leprosy and tuberculoid leprosy lying at the two ends of a wide spectrum of disease.

Leprosy is widely prevalent in India. It is endemic in Bihar, Jharkhand, Chhattisgarh, U.P., West Bengal and M.P.

Source of Infection

1. Droplet Infection

Leprosy spreads via aerosols containing the organism.

2. Contact transmission

It can be transmitted from person to person by close contact between an infectious patient and a healthy person.

Signs and Symptoms

One or more of the following cardinal features clinically characterizes leprosy:

1. Hypo pigmented patches.
2. Partial or total loss of cutaneous sensations in affected areas.
3. Presence of thickened nerves.
4. Presence of AFB in the skin/nasal smears

The signs of advanced disease are:

Presence of nodules/lumps especially in the skin of the face and ears, plantar ulcers, loss of fingers/toes, nasal depression, foot drop, claw toes and other deformities.

Diagnosis

Criteria for diagnosis of leprosy are:

1. Hypo pigmented or reddish skin lesion(s) with definite loss of sensation.
2. Involvement of peripheral nerves.
3. Demonstration of organism in the lesions.

The first two cardinal signs can be identified by clinical examination alone while the third can be identified by examination of the slit skin smear. At least one of the above three criteria must be present for the diagnosis of leprosy.

The organisms can be demonstrated in skin by following methods:

Skin smears—from both ear lobes.

Nasal smears or blows—best prepared from early morning mucous material.

Nasal scrapings

Footpad culture—organism cultured in footpad of mice.

Indirect Tests

Histamine test—Recommended when difficulty is experienced in the diagnosis.

Biopsy—when the examination detailed above does not yield the diagnosis, histopathology may be necessary. It allows classification of the disease and also gives information about the bacterial content of disease.

Immunological Tests

Tests for detecting cell-mediated immunity are: Lepromin test, Lymphocyte transformation test (LTT), Leucocyte migration inhibition test (LMIT).

Tests for detecting humoral immunity: Fluorescent leprosy antibody absorption test, ELISA.

II. Viral Diseases

AIDS

This is a fatal illness caused by HIV, which breaks

down the body's immune system leaving the victim vulnerable to a variety of life threatening opportunistic infections.

In India, 39,742 cases of AIDS have been reported to WHO up to 31st Oct. 2002. This includes 29,907 males and 9,835 females. Migration both within and between the states is a potential source of spread of disease. The most commonly affected states are Maharashtra, Manipur, and Tamil Nadu.

Source of Infection

1. *Sexual transmission*—Through heterosexual, homosexual and bisexual routes.
2. *Parenteral route*—via contaminated needles and other skin piercing instruments.
3. Through transfusion of contaminated blood and blood products.
4. Transplacentally or perinatally from HIV infected female to her newborn baby.

Diagnosis

An adult or adolescent (> 12 years of age) is considered to have AIDS if at least 2 of the following major signs are present in combination with at least one of the minor signs.

Major Signs

1. Weight loss > 10% of body weight.
2. Chronic diarrhoea for > 1 month.
3. Prolonged fever for > 1 month (intermittent/ constant).

Minor Signs

- ❑ Persistent cough for > 1 month.
- ❑ Generalized pruritic dermatitis.
- ❑ History of Herpes zoster.
- ❑ Oropharyngeal candidiasis.

- Chronic progressive disseminated Herpes simplex infection.
- Generalized lymphadenopathy.

Laboratory Diagnosis

The laboratory diagnosis of HIV infection is usually made by demonstrating specific anti-HIV antibodies in the blood of an individual. These antibodies appear in the blood within 6 months in 99% cases.

1. ELISA Test

It is a highly sensitive test. Its low cost, need for small serum sample, commercial availability and good reproducibility make it a widely used test.

2. Western Blot Test

This test has higher specificity. Confirmation of an ELISA positive sample is usually done with Western blot test. It is much more expensive than ELISA.

3. PCR

It is useful for an early diagnosis. This is also an expensive test.

4. Virus Culture

This type of testing is very expensive and requires extensive laboratory support.

Viral Hepatitis

Viral hepatitis is infection of the liver caused by any of the following 6 viruses:

A, B, C, D, E, G—Hepatitis A and E mainly spread through fecal-oral route, usually through water. The other four are usually transmitted parenterally; of these B and C types are most dangerous and type B is the most common.

Hepatitis is widely prevalent in India. Hepatitis A virus causes a relatively benign disease and does not constitute a major public health problem in India. In contrast, hepatitis B is responsible for severe liver damage and is associated with chronic liver disease and hepatocellular carcinoma. Hepatitis virus non-A non-B consists of at least 2 viruses: one that is parenterally transmitted like hepatitis B virus, i.e. hepatitis C and the other is hepatitis E transmitted through fecal oral route like hepatitis A virus.

It has been estimated that approximately 4 million people in India suffer every year from one or the other form of acute viral hepatitis

Source of Infection

1. Fecal oral—Hepatitis A, E.
2. Parenteral and sexual transmission—Hepatitis B and C.

Signs and Symptoms

Jaundice, fever, loss of appetite, malaise, high coloured urine.

Diagnosis

A specific laboratory diagnosis can be obtained by the following:

Hepatitis A

1. Demonstration of HAV particle or specific viral antigen in the faeces.
2. Demonstration of a rise in anti-HAV titre.
3. Detection of IBM antibodies to HAV in the patient's serum.

Hepatitis B

Serologic diagnosis of acute HBV infection requires assays for HbsAg and IgM anti HBC.

Prevention

The best means of reducing the spread of infection is by simple measures, e.g.—

- ❑ Hand-washing before eating and after toilet.
- ❑ Drinking filtered clean water.

- Proper autoclaving of syringes, nèedles and other equipment.
- Avoid spilling blood during collection, storage and transport.
- Blood donors should be screened for HBV infection.

Severe Acute Respiratory Syndrome (SARS)

A new disease called severe acute respiratory syndrome (SARS) is a respiratory illness that has recently been reported in Asia, North America and Europe. The new corona virus is the leading hypothesis for the cause of SARS.

Mode of Transmission

The primary way that SARS appears to spread is by close person-to-person contact. Most cases of SARS have involved people who cared for or lived with someone with SARS, or had direct contact with infectious material (for example, respiratory secretions) from a person who has SARS. Potential ways in which SARS can be spread include touching the skin of other people or objects that are contaminated with infectious droplets and then touching your eye(s), nose, or mouth. This can happen when someone who is sick with SARS coughs or sneezes droplets onto themselves, other people, or nearby surfaces.

Symptoms of SARS

In general, SARS begins with a fever greater than 100.4°F [>38.0°C]. Other symptoms may include headache, an overall feeling of discomfort, and body aches. Some people also experience mild respiratory symptoms. After 2 to 7 days, SARS patients may develop a dry cough and have trouble breathing.

Diagnosis

Non-specific tests

- Chest X-Rays,
- Blood cultures,

- ❑ Sputum Gram's stain and culture, and
- ❑ Pulse oximetry.

Specific Tests for SARS

1. Molecular tests (PCR)

Polymerase chain reaction (PCR) can detect genetic material of the SARS-Corona Virus (CoV) in various specimens (blood, stool, respiratory secretions or body tissues). Principally, existing PCR tests are very specific but lack sensitivity. This means that negative tests cannot rule out the presence of the SARS virus in patients.

2. Antibody tests

These tests detect antibodies produced in response to the SARS corona virus infection. Different types of antibodies (IgM and IgG) appear and change in level during the course of infection. They can be undetectable at the early stage of infection. IgG usually remains detectable after resolution of the illness.

The following test formats are being developed:

- ❑ *ELISA*: a test detecting a mixture of IgM and IgG antibodies in the serum of SARS patients yields positive results reliably at around day 21 after the onset of illness.
- ❑ *IFA (Immunofluorescence Assay)*: a test detecting IgM antibodies in serum of SARS patients yields positive results after about day 10 of illness. This test format is also used to test for IgG.

Positive antibody test results: Indicate a previous infection with SARS-CoV. Seroconversion from negative to positive or a four-fold rise in antibody titre from acute to convalescent serum indicates recent infection.

Negative antibody test results: No detection of antibody after 21 days from onset of illness seems to indicate that no infection with SARS-CoV took place.

3. Cell culture

Virus in specimens (such as respiratory secretions, blood or stool) from SARS patients can also be detected by inoculating cell cultures and growing the virus. Once isolated, the virus must be identified as the SARS virus with further tests.

Positive cell culture results indicate the presence of live SARS-CoV in the sample tested.

Negative cell culture results do not exclude SARS.

III. Parasitic Diseases

Malaria

This is a disease transmitted to man by certain species of infected female Anopheles mosquito. It is clinically characterized by episodes of chills and fever, enlargement of spleen and anemia. The incidence of malaria in India is about 2 million cases per year.

Agent

About 70% of the infections are reported to be due to Plasmodium vivax, 25-30% due to Plasmodium falciparum and 4-8% due to mixed infection. Plasmodium falciparum gives rise to a series of phenomena which if not effectively treated threatens the life of the patient in 1-3 days.

Life History

The malarial parasite undergoes two cycles of development:

The Human (asexual) Cycle

After passing through a developmental phase in liver cells it resides in RBCs and are carried by circulating blood to all organs.

The mosquito cycle

The sexual cycle of parasite occurs in female Anopheles mosquito.

Reservoir of Infection

A human reservoir is one who harbors the sexual forms gametocytes of the parasite. There exists no other animal reservoir of human plasmodium except chimpanzees in tropical Africa.

Vector

The female Anopheles mosquito is the vector in malarial transmission. Out of about 45 species of Anopheles mosquito in India only a few are regarded as vectors of primary importance.

Mode of Transmission

1. The female anopheles mosquito acts as intermediary in transmitting infection to man. During the act of biting the mosquito pierces the skin and the salivary secretions are injected into the punctured wound.
2. *Transfusion malaria*—When infected persons are used as donors.
3. *Congenital malaria*—Transfusion of malaria in fetus in utero through some placental defect.
4. *Malaria in drug addicts*—Through use of same syringe when one of them is infected.

Signs and Symptoms

- *Febrile paroxysm*—Fever with chills and rigors occurs after an interval of 24 hours in P. vivax and 48 hours in P. falciparum.
- *Anemia*—Due to breaking down of RBCs.
- *Splenic enlargement*—This is one of the most important physical signs in malaria.

Laboratory Diagnosis and Control of Malaria

Malaria being a public health problem of great significance; the government of India aims to control this disease on a priority. Surveillance is a key element in the National Malaria eradication programme and involves timely collection and examination of blood smears.

Blood Film

Microscopic examination of blood film forms one of the most important diagnostic procedures in malaria. A thick and a thin film are prepared at the same time. The parasite is quickly detected in the thick film and the thin film examined for identifying the species.

There may be difficulties in detecting the malarial parasite when—

- Sample is taken after anti-malarial drug.
- Sample is taken during afebrile interval especially in falciparum malaria.
- In cases of primary infection during the first 2-3 days.

Blood Counts

Serological tests

- Indirect haemagglutination test.
- Immunofluorescence test.

Treatment

Chloroquin is the mainstay of treatment, when chloroquin resistant malaria is encountered—sulfodoxine, pyrimethamine and primaquin are used. While drugs may provide relief, the ultimate solution lies in interruption of transmission.

Leishmaniasis

This parasite of the genus leishmania causes Kala azar (visceral leishmaniasis) and oriental store (cutaneous leishmaniasis). Patients with Kala azar have intermittent fever anemia, loss of weight and enlargement of spleen. It is endemic in many parts of India: it is especially common in Assam, Bengal, Bihar, Orissa and eastern U.P. Kala azar is transmitted by the bite of the sand fly.

Life cycle

The parasite exists in two stages:

1. *Amastigote form*—occurs in man.
2. *Promastigote form*—occurs in the gut of sand fly.

Reservoir of Infection

In India man is the main and only source of infection.

Mode of Transmission

The infection is transmitted to man by the bite of an infected sand fly which in order to take a blood meal liberates the organism into the wound.

Signs and Symptoms

- ❑ *Fever*—continuous/remittent type.
- ❑ *Splenic enlargement*—may be massive.
- ❑ Liver enlargement.
- ❑ Anemia.

Lab Diagnosis

1. Direct evidence

- ❑ Thick blood film.
- ❑ Blood culture.
- ❑ *Splenic puncture*—When spleen is considerably enlarged it is one of the most valuable method of establishing a diagnosis.
- ❑ *Bone marrow biopsy*—This is a certain method of diagnosis of Kala azar.

2. Indirect evidence

- ❑ *Blood counts*—marked decrease in neutrophils.
- ❑ *Serological test*—rise in gamma globulin detected by aldehyde and antimony test.
  —Complement fixation test.
- ❑ *Skin test*—indicates delayed hypersensitivity to

leishmania antigen and is useful to identify groups at risk of infection

Filariasis

This is a major public health problem in India and is caused by a nematode worm. In India it is chiefly along the sea coast and along the banks of big rivers.

Life Cycle

The parasite passes its life cycle in two hosts:

1. Man
2. Mosquito

Mode of Transmission

It is transmitted by the bite of infective mosquitoes; the main vectors in India are the culex and mansonia mosquitoes.

Signs and Symptoms

The disease manifestations are of two types:

1. *Lymphatic filariasis*—fever, lymphadenitis, lymphangitis and epididymoorchitis. In chronic diseases there may be localized elephantiasis of legs, scrotum, penis, arm, vulva etc.
2. In occult filariasis as in tropical pulmonary eosinophilia—microfilariae are not found in the blood and the clinical manifestations are due to hypersensitivity to filarial antigens.

Laboratory Diagnosis

Direct Evidence

1. Thick film made at night with capillary blood is examined for microfilariae.
2. *Membrane filter concentration*: Venous blood is sampled and large volume is filtered to detect low-density carriers.
3. *DEC provocation test*: In this test, the blood is

examined one hour after administration of DEC which induces microfilaria to appear in blood

Indirect Evidence

- ❑ Increased eosinophils in blood.
- ❑ Intradermal test.

Serological test using immunofluorescent and complement fixing technique.

Anemias

According to WHO expert group, anemia should be considered to exist when Hb is below 13g% in males, 12g% in non-pregnant female and 11% in pregnant female.

Iron Deficiency Anemia

Iron deficiency anemia—This is most common cause of anemia. It is common in infancy and women of child-bearing age. According to WHO estimates, the prevalence of nutritional anemia in India is 76% in pre-school children, 50% in school children, 50-80% in women and 70-90% in pregnant women. Its effects range from simple depletion of iron stores to severe iron deficiency. Iron deficiency can occur either because of excessive body loss or because of inadequate intake of iron.

	Megaloblastic anemia due to folate deficiency	*Megaloblastic anemia due to vitamin B12 deficiency*
Decreased intake	Nutritional deficiency (more in vegetarians)	Nutritional deficiency (more in non-vegetarians)
Impaired absorption	Celiac disease Tropical sprue	Pernicious anemia Gastrectomy Celiac disease Tropical sprue
Increased demand	Pregnancy/puerparium Carcinoma Leukemias	Fish tapeworm infestation

Causes

Chronic blood loss

- *Menstrual blood loss*—related to pregnancy and delivery.
- *GI Blood loss*—Occult blood loss from GIT (peptic ulcer, piles, cancer, parasites, e.g. hook worm infestation) may go undetected until patients present with symptoms of anemia.

Increased iron requirement

- Infancy, adolescence.
- Pregnancy and lactation.

Iron malabsorption

- In certain malabsorption syndromes.

Inadequate iron intake

- The poor food quality and largely vegetarian diets in developing countries may result in iron deficiency.

Signs and Symptoms

- Non-specific symptoms include fatigue, weakness, shortness of breath.
- Oral lesions, e.g. soreness and cracking in the corners of the lips, soreness of tongue and mouth.
- Difficulty in swallowing.
- Flattened and thinned nails.
- Compulsive ingestion of clay, paint, etc.

Diagnosis

- *Decreased hemoglobin*—Values below those given in definition indicate anemia.
- *Peripheral blood smear*—Microcytic hypochromic anemia.

- Blood indices.
- *Serum iron studies*—This is more useful index than hemoglobin concentration.
- *Serum ferritin*—The single most sensitive tool for evaluating iron status is by measurement of serum ferritn. It reflects the size of iron stores in body.

Megaloblastic Anemia

This occurs due to deficiency of either folic acid or vitamin B12. In India, folate deficiency due to a combination of inadequate intake and malabsorption is the cause of most cases, vitamin B12 deficiency being less prevalent. The higher incidence of nutritional folate as compared to vitamin B12 deficiency is related to the smaller body stores of folate and the greater liability of folate to destruction on cooking.

Causes

Signs and Symptoms

- Fatigue, weakness, shortness of breath.
- Glossitis—beefy, red sore tongue and angular stomatitis.
- Peripheral neuropathy.

Diagnosis

1. Macrocytic anemia.
2. (a) Folate deficiency:
   - (i) Low serum levels of Folic acid,
   - (ii) red cell folate assays.

   (b) Vitamin B12 deficiency:
   - (i) Serum B12 assay: microbiological assay, Radioisotope assay,
   - (ii) Radioactive B12 absorption test, i.e. Schilling test.
3. Bone marrow examination.

Leukemias

Leukemias are diseases in which abnormal proliferation

of hemopoietic cells causes progressively increasing infiltration of the bone marrow. Leukemias account for about 4-5% of cancers among all age groups but is the most common malignancy in children. The overall incidence is roughly 3-5/100,000 people per year.

Major clinical forms observed are:

- Acute myeloblastic leukemia (AML).
- Acute lymphoblastic leukemia (ALL).
- Chronic myeloid leukemia (CML).
- Chronic lymphocytic leukemia (CLL).

There is male preponderance of roughly in the ratio of 1.4:1.1. AML is much more common in adults than in children. ALL comprises 75-80% of childhood acute leukemias. In majority of the cases, CLL is detected between 45-75 years of age.

Signs and Symptoms

Acute Leukemias

- Fatigue, weight loss, weakness.
- Enlargement of liver and spleen.
- Enlargement of lymph nodes.
- Bone pains.
- Predisposition to infections.
- Easy bruisability.

Chronic Leukemias

- Enlargement of liver and spleen.
- Enlargement of lymph nodes in CLL.

Diagnosis of Leukemias

- Peripheral blood examination.
- Bone marrow examination.

In conclusion, disease control requires all the measures to reduce the incidence, prevalence and consequence of an illness. Early detection and prompt treatment can reduce both the incidence and mortality related to a disease.

6

Let Your Heart be Fit: Pros and Cons of Primary and Secondary Prevention of Heart Failure

I. INTRODUCTION

Heart failure is not the end of the road. Contrary to usual belief, its primary and secondary prevention is possible. Uncared it can lead to disability and death due to sub-optimal functioning of the heart. Congestive Heart Failure (CHF) or heart failure (HF) usually develops gradually. It is a condition in which the heart does not pump blood to different parts of the body, as well, as it should. The body does not get the right amount of blood and oxygen it needs to work properly. The weakened pumping action can cause a back-up stagnation of fluid in the lungs and other parts of the body. Without a proper oxygen supply and with congestion, you may feel tired and short of breath. It does not entail complete stoppage of the heart to function. It denotes relative insufficiency. It usually develops slowly, often over years. The heart keeps pumping, but not as efficiently as a healthy heart. The severity of the condition determines the impact it has on a person's life. At one end of the spectrum, the mild form of heart failure may have little or no effect on a person's life; at the other end, severe heart failure can interfere with even simple activities and can prove even fatal. But all forms of heart failure, even the mildest, are a serious health problem, which must be treated. The palliative care approach should concentrate on quality of life and good symptom control, a whole-person approach, to patients and their careers, and respect patient's autonomy and choice.

1.1 Underlying Heart Problem

Heart failure may result from any of the following: heart valve disease—caused by past rheumatic fever or other infections, high blood pressure (hypertension, infections of the heart valves and/or heart muscle (i.e., endocarditis), previous heart attack(s) (myocardial infarction)—scar tissue from previous attacks may interfere with the heart muscle's ability to work normally, coronary artery disease—narrowed arteries that supply blood to the heart muscle, cardiomyopathy—a disease of the heart muscle, congenital heart disease/defects (present at birth), cardiac arrhythmias (irregular heartbeats), chronic lung disease and pulmonary embolism, drug-induced heart failure, excessive sodium intake, hemorrhage and anemia.

1.2 Fluid Retention

Heart failure interferes with the kidney's normal function of eliminating excess sodium and waste from the ody. In heart failure, the body retains more fluid—resulting in swelling of the ankles and legs. Fluid may also collect in the lungs—resulting in shortness of breath. Other Symptoms may include: weight gain, visible swelling of the legs and ankles, fatigue, loss of appetite, nausea, and persistent cough. The severity of the condition and symptoms depends on how much of the heart's pumping capacity has been lost.

1.3 Types of Heart Failure?

Systolic heart failure: This occurs when the heart's ability to contract decreases. The heart cannot pump with enough force to push sufficient amount of blood into the circulation. Blood coming into the heart from the lungs may back up and cause fluid to leak into the lungs, a condition known as pulmonary congestion. Diastolic heart failure occurs when the heart has a problem in relaxing. The heart cannot properly fill with blood because the muscle has become stiff, losing its ability to relax. This form may lead to fluid accumulation, especially in the feet, ankles and legs. Some patients may have lung congestion.

1.4 How Common is Heart Failure?

In India it is one of the common conditions of disability and death. The condition is slightly more common among men than women and is twice as common among blacks as compared to whites. In a sense, heart failure's growing presence as a health problem reflects the Nation's changing population: More people are living longer. People aged 65 and older represent the fastest growing segment of the population, and the risk of heart failure increases with age. The condition affects 1 percent of people aged 50, but about 5 percent of people aged 75.

2. WHAT CAUSES HEART FAILURE?

As stated above, the heart loses some of its blood-pumping ability as a natural consequence of ageing. However, a number of other factors can lead to a potentially life-threatening loss of pumping activity. As said above, it is generally a symptom of another heart disease. Heart failure is closely associated with the major risk factors for coronary heart disease: smoking, high cholesterol levels, hypertension (persistent high blood pressure), diabetes and abnormal blood sugar levels and obesity. A person can change or eliminate those risk factors and thus lower their risk of developing or aggravating their heart disease and heart failure. Among prominent risk factors, hypertension (high blood pressure) and diabetes are particularly important. Uncontrolled high blood pressure increases the risk of heart failure by 200 percent, compared with those who do not have hypertension. Moreover, the degree of risk appears directly related to the severity of the high blood pressure. Persons with diabetes have about a two to eight-fold greater risk of heart failure than those without diabetes. Women with diabetes have a greater risk of heart failure than men with diabetes. Higher risk comes from diabetes' association with other heart failure risk factors, such as high blood pressure, obesity, and high cholesterol levels. However, the disease process in diabetes also damages the heart muscle. The presence of coronary disease is among the greatest risks for heart failure. Muscle damage and scarring caused by a heart attack greatly increases the risk of heart failure. Cardiac arrhythmias, or irregular heartbeats, also raise heart failure risk. Any disorder that causes abnormal swelling or thickening of the heart sets the stage for heart failure. In some people, heart failure arises from problems with heart valves, the flap-like structures that help regulate blood flow through the heart. Infections in the heart are another source of increased risk for heart failure. A single risk factor may be sufficient to cause heart failure, but a combination of factors increases the risk. Advanced age adds to the potential impact of any heart failure risk.

3. WHAT ARE THE SYMPTOMS?

Perhaps the best-known symptom is shortness of breath ("dyspnea"). In heart failure, this may result from excess fluid in the lungs. The breathing difficulties may occur at rest or during exercise. In some cases, congestion may be severe enough to prevent or interrupt sleep. Fatigue or easy tiring is another common symptom. As the heart's pumping capacity decreases, muscles and other tissues receive less oxygen and nutrition, which are carried in the blood. Without proper "fuel," the body cannot perform as much work, which translates into fatigue. Fluid accumulation, or edema, may cause swelling of the feet, ankles, legs, and occasionally, the abdomen. Excess fluid retained by the body may result in weight gain, which sometimes occurs fairly quickly. Persistent coughing is another common sign, especially coughing that regularly produces mucus or pink, blood-tinged sputum. Some people develop difficult breathing or wheezing. Depression occurs in about one-third of patients and it frequently goes unrecognized. Other severe common symptoms are sleep disturbance and nausea and vomiting. Distressing pain is common throughout the last year of life and at around the time of death. In addition, patients often experience confusion and short-term memory loss.

3.1 Develops Slowly

Because heart failure usually develops slowly, the symptoms may not appear until the condition has progressed over years. The heart hides the underlying problem by making adjustments that delay—but do not prevent—the eventual loss in pumping capacity. The heart adjusts, or compensates, in three ways to cope with and hide the effects of heart failure:

- Enlargement ("dilatation"), which allows more blood into the heart;
- Thickening of muscle fibers ("hypertrophy") to strengthen the heart muscle, which allows the heart to contract more forcefully and pump more blood; and
- More frequent contraction, which increases circulation.

By making these adjustments, or compensating, the heart can temporarily make up for losses in pumping ability, sometimes for years. However, compensation has its limits.

3.2 Shortness of Breath

Shortness of breath is caused by fluid build-up in the lungs. You may:

- Feel as though you are not getting enough air;
- Have problems breathing when you lie flat;
- Feel more out of breath when you exert yourself or exercise; and
- Have a dry hacking cough or be unable to catch your breath at night or wake up in the middle of the night short of breath.

3.3 Swollen Ankles and Legs

Swollen ankles and legs happen because there is too much fluid in the tissues of your body. This is known as edema. You may notice that:

- your shoes are tighter; and
- You have more swelling in your feet and legs in the evening.

3.4 Sudden Weight Gain

Sudden weight gain occurs when your kidneys save extra water and salt because of sluggish circulation. This extra water is translated into a gain in body weight. You may notice that:

- Rings on your fingers feel smaller;
- your shoes or clothes feel tighter; and
- your waist belt feels tighter.

3.5 Tiredness/Loss of Energy

Tiredness and/or loss of energy are due to slow removal of waste products from your body and slow delivery of oxygen to muscles. You may:

- Tire more easily; and
- Need more rest periods during the day.

3.6 Loss/Change in Appetite

Loss or change in appetite happens when your body has less energy to digest food and there is too much fluid in your tissues. You may feel:

- Bloated after eating very little; and
- Nausea, with abdominal pain and/or tenderness.

Factors that increase symptoms are:

- High salt foods or beverages;
- Medications that cause salt and water to be retained;
- Fast heart rhythms;
- Cold or flu; and
- Excessive fluid intake.

4. HOW DO DOCTORS DIAGNOSE HEART FAILURE?

In many cases, physicians diagnose heart failure during a physical examination. Readily identifiable signs are shortness of breath, fatigue, and swollen ankles and feet. The physician also will check for the presence of risk factors, such as hypertension, obesity, and a history of heart problems. Using a stethoscope, the physician can listen to a patient's breath and identify the sounds of lung congestion. The stethoscope also picks up the abnormal heart sounds indicative of heart failure. In addition to a complete medical history and physical examination, diagnostic procedures for congestive heart failure may include any, or a combination of, the following: laboratory tests, electrocardiogram (ECG or EKG)—a test that records the electrical activity of the heart, shows abnormal rhythms (arrhythmias or dysrhythmias), and detects heart muscle damage. Chest X-ray, echocardiogram (also known as echo)—a non-invasive test that uses sound waves to produce a study of the motion of the heart's chambers and valves. The echo sound waves create an image on the monitor as an ultrasound transducer is passed over the heart.

5. WHAT TREATMENTS ARE AVAILABLE?

Heart failure caused by an excessive workload is curable by treating the primary disease, such as anemia or thyrotoxicosis. Also curable are forms caused by anatomical problems, such as a heart valve defect. These defects can be surgically corrected. However, for the common forms of heart failure—due to damaged heart muscle—no known cure exists. But treatment for these forms may be successful. The treatment seeks to improve patients' quality of life and length of survival through lifestyle change and drug therapy. Patients can minimize the effects of heart failure by controlling the risk factors for heart disease. Obvious steps include quit smoking, lose weight if necessary, abstaining from alcohol, and making dietary changes to reduce the amount of salt and fat consumed. Regular, modest exercise is helpful for many patients, though a physician should carefully monitor the amount and intensity. But, even with lifestyle changes, most heart failure patients require medication. Many patients receive two or more drugs. Specific treatment will be determined by your physician(s) based on: your age, overall health, and medical history, extent of the disease, your tolerance for specific medications, procedures, or therapies, expectations for the course of the disease, your opinion or preference. If the heart failure is caused by a valve disorder, then surgery is usually required. If a disease, such as anemia causes the heart failure then the disease is treated. And, although there is no cure for heart failure due to a damaged heart muscle, many forms of treatment prove successful. The goal of treatment is to improve a person's quality of life by making the appropriate lifestyle changes and implementing drug therapy.

Several types of drugs have proven useful in the treatment of heart failure:

- Diuretics help reduce the amount of fluid in the body and are useful for patients with fluid retention and hypertension.
- Digitalis increases the force of the heart's contractions, helping to improve circulation.
- Results of recent studies have placed more emphasis on the use of drugs known as angiotensin converting enzyme (ACE) inhibitors. Several large studies have indicated that ACE inhibitors improve survival among heart failure patients and may slow, or perhaps even prevent, the loss of heart pumping activity.

Originally developed as a treatment for hypertension, ACE inhibitors help heart failure patients by decreasing the pressure inside blood vessels. As a result, the heart does not have to work as hard to pump blood through the vessels. Patients who cannot take ACE inhibitors may get a nitrate and/or a drug called hydralazine, each of which helps relax tension in blood vessels and improves blood flow. Sometimes, heart failure is life threatening. Usually, this happens when drug therapy and lifestyle changes fail to control its symptoms. In such cases, a heart transplant may be the only treatment option. However, candidates for transplantation often have to wait months or even years before a suitable donor heart is found. Recent studies indicate that some transplant candidates improve during this waiting period through drug treatment and other therapy, and can be removed from the transplant list. Transplant candidates who do not improve sometimes need mechanical pumps, which are attached to the heart. Called left ventricular assist devices (LVAD), the machines take over part or virtually all of the heart's blood-pumping activity. However, current LVAD are not permanent solutions for heart failure but are considered bridges to transplantation. An experimental surgical procedure for severe heart failure is available at a few U.S. medical centers. The procedure, called cardiomyoplasty, involves detaching one end of a muscle in the back, wrapping it around the heart, and then suturing the muscle to the heart. An implanted electric stimulator causes the back muscle to contract, pumping blood from the heart.

Let us study some of the non-medication options in the lifestyle.

5.1 Managing Fluid Build-up

- ❑ Do breathing exercises regularly: Slowly breathe in and blow slowly out through your mouth. Repeat 2-3 times. Do a few of these each hour that you are awake. These breathing exercises will help keep your lungs clear.
- ❑ A strong cough is important to clear lung secretions and phlegm;
- ❑ Try support stockings to help reduce leg swelling;
- ❑ Raise your legs when resting;
- ❑ Use a foot stool when sitting;
- ❑ When sleeping, raise the head of the bed 4 to 6 inches, or use a wedge shaped pillow under the mattress, or use a reclining chair at night time.
- ❑ Record your weight in a diary to show to your healthcare team.

5.2 Weigh yourself Regularly

Fluid build-up in your body shows on your scale as weight gain. A sudden weight gain when you have been eating normally may be an early sign of fluid build-up. If your weight increases more than 2 pounds (1 kg) in 2 days, or 5 pounds (3 kg) in a single week, call your nurse or doctor. Weigh yourself 3 times a week.

5.3 Know about Alcohol

The Heart Foundation recommends that you drink no more than one to two drinks per day. If you drink alcohol, you may have to severely reduce your intake of other drinks. You may have to abstain from alcohol completely, since alcohol impairs heart function. One drink is equal to:

- ❑ 1 bottle of beer (12 oz./350 mL/5% alcohol), or
- ❑ 1 glass of wine (5 oz./150 mL/12% alcohol), or
- ❑ 1 mixed drink (1 ½ oz./150 mL/40% alcohol).

You need to discuss drinking alcohol with your doctor because: Alcohol may change how your medication works; Alcohol can affect other medical conditions you may have; Alcohol suppresses heart function; Alcohol may provoke potentially lethal irregular heart rhythms.

5.4 Be Smoke Free

Smoking, or exposure to second-hand smoke, makes the heart work harder and decreases the amount of oxygen carried in the blood. Nicotine injures the lining of the arteries and increases the build-up of fat deposits in that area.

5.5 Balance Activity

It is important to balance your daily activities with rest periods to help control your symptoms. Some people find if they are too active one day, they are very tired for the next few days. Taking rest periods during the day is helpful. Rest and activity . . . a matter of balance. Complete prolonged bed rest, which is contained in old textbooks, is no longer recommended. Here are some suggestions to help you balance activity and rest:

- ❑ Plan ahead;
- ❑ Make-up a schedule of activities for the day and week. Include rest periods in your schedule;
- ❑ Set priorities. Do the most important job first;
- ❑ Alternate heavy and light tasks throughout the day and week;
- ❑ Sit while working when possible and keep items within easy reach; and
- ❑ Work at a comfortable pace.

Physical Activity

Participate in regular physical activity—

- ❑ Regular physical activity may help you to feel better and make your daily activities easier;
- ❑ Physical activity does not have to be hard to be valuable. The amount of work the heart does varies depending on how you feel;
- ❑ Walking is one of the best activities for improving your health;
- ❑ A healthcare team member can advise you about the right kind and amount of activity for you;
- ❑ The following activities are not recommended because they may cause your heart to work harder than it should:
  - Competitive or contact sports;
  - Activities that demand sudden bursts of energy such as baseball, hockey, etc.;
  - Exercises that make you hold your breath or bear down; and
  - Activities that require you to lift your own weight (pull-ups) or other weight.

5.6 Walking Guidelines

- ❑ Discuss your walking plan with a healthcare team member;
- ❑ If you are unusually tired or feel ill, don't walk;
- ❑ Walk before meals or 90 minutes gap after a meal;
- ❑ Walk on level surfaces, and avoid hills;

- ❑ Walk in a familiar area;
- ❑ Walking in hot and humid or cold and windy weather may increase your CHF. You may want to walk indoors (e.g., inside a shopping mall) if you:
    - Become short of breath;
    - Feel weak, tired or dizzy;
    - Have any discomfort; and
    - Have a fast heart rate.

Walking Program

Below is a suggested walking program, but remember to ask your doctor what would be the best for you.

Week 1 to 2: Walk 5 to 10 minutes;
Week 3 to 4: Walk 10 to 15 minutes;
Week 5 to 6: Walk 15 to 20 minutes; and
Week 7 to 8: Walk 20 to 30 minutes.

- ❑ Aim to walk three times per week;
- ❑ You should be back to your pre-walk, or resting state, within 10 to 15 minutes of completing your exercise. If not, the next time you exercise, cut the distance you walk in half; and
- ❑ Stop and go back to the previous level of activity if you develop any symptoms. Listen to what your body is telling you. You may be trying to do too much.

5.7 Work

You may have concerns about whether you can continue to work full-time or part-time outside the home. This will depend on your symptoms and the type of job you have. Concerns about finances or retraining may also be bothering you. If you are a homemaker, you may also need to take time off. Ask family members, friends and neighbours for help. Talk to your doctor and study awareness pamphlets.

5.8 Intimate Relations

You and your partner may experience anxiety about

sexual activity. This is very common. Intercourse with your partner is not as hard on your heart as you may think. Research shows that sexual activity takes about the same energy as walking up two flights of stairs or walking briskly. Foreplay is a good warm-up for the increased activity of intercourse. This may be a time when you desire sex less. Some reasons may be:

- Medications;
- Fatigue; and
- Stress.

5.9 Stress

Stress is often a productive part of everyday life. But when stress becomes "distress", it makes your heart work harder. Although stress cannot be eliminated, it can be managed:

- Learn what triggers stress for you;
- Learn to recognize your symptoms when stressed;
- Set aside time to relax every day;
- Try relaxation techniques and stress management programs;
- Get support from family and friends;
- Talk about your problems;
- Manage stress with regular physical activity; and
- Seek professional help if stress becomes too overwhelming.

5.10 Cold and Flu

- Avoid coming in contact with people who have colds or the flu; and
- Get a flu shot every autumn.

5.11 Sharing Feelings

When you were diagnosed with CHF, you may have felt shock, anger, fear, anxiety, loss, or sadness. This is expected. Your family and friends may have felt the same way. Sharing your feelings with each other is one way of coping with the changes that are happening. You will need each other for support as you start to look ahead to the future.

6. MEDICATION TIPS

- ❑ Follow the directions for your prescriptions carefully. Medications will work only if you use them correctly;
- ❑ Take your medication regularly, even if you feel well;
- ❑ Take your medications at the same time or times everyday;
- ❑ Keep these and all prescription drugs out of the reach of children;
- ❑ If you forget to take your medication don't double the next dose. Call your doctor or pharmacist for advice;
- ❑ Medications have many different actions and side effects. Call your doctor, nurse or pharmacist if you have questions, or if you notice side effects;
- ❑ When you take these medications, your doctor may request blood tests. These tests check the health of your kidneys and the levels of sodium and potassium in your blood;
- ❑ Bring all your medications with you when seeing any doctor. It is important for the doctor to know what medication you are already taking. There may be changes in your prescriptions because of interactions between medications;
- ❑ Make sure you have enough medication to last until your next prescription refill. Many pharmacies will deliver medications;
- ❑ Carry a wallet card that lists all your medications, doses and times taken. Your pharmacist or nurse can help you make this list; and
- ❑ When traveling, keep your medication with you in a carry-on bag. Never pack your medication in checked luggage. Be sure your medication is properly labeled and in its original container.

7. COMMON MEDICATIONS

There are five types of medications most commonly used to treat CHF. These are:

- Aldosterone antagonists;
- Angiotensin Converting Enzyme (ACE) inhibitors;
- Beta blockers;
- Digoxin; and
- Diuretics.

You may not need all of these medications, depending on your type of CHF and your degree of symptoms. Each of these groups may encompass several different drugs. You may need one or more drugs from each group. It is important to understand how they work together and what they can do for you.

7.1 Aldosterone Antagonists

These reduce the stress on the heart and also have a weak diuretic effect. The only drug of this class that is currently available for general use is spironolactone. The use of this drug is usually limited to patients with advanced disease and severe symptoms. Spironolactone is usually taken once a day. Before this medication is prescribed, your doctor will need to check your kidney function and blood potassium level. Some of your other medications may need to be adjusted as well. Some side effects you might experience are:

- Too much potassium in the body. This will occur especially in patients with impaired kidney function. Close monitoring of blood potassium levels is therefore necessary.
- Gynecomastia or enlargement of the breasts in males. Occasionally this would require the discontinuation of the medication.

7.2 ACE Inhibitors

These prevent the production of a chemical that causes blood vessels to narrow. As a result, blood pressure drops and the heart does not have to work hard to pump blood. This medication will help reduce the stress on your heart and may prevent your symptoms from becoming worse. Take this medication at a convenient time every day. How many times a day you take your medication, and whether you should take it with food will depend upon which drug you are prescribed. You may not feel differently immediately after starting to take this medication, but it is important to continue to take it. Some side effects you might experience are:

- Weakness, dizziness or light headedness;
- Skin rash;
- Dry cough;
- Swelling of the face, neck, tongue, hands or feet;
- Altered taste;
- Persistent dry cough;
- Diarrhea;
- Difficulty breathing; and
- Yellowed eyes or skin.

Seek medical help immediately if you experience swelling of the face, tongue, hands or feet.

7.3 Beta Blockers

Beta-blockers protect the heart and prolong the patient's life. Some patients may initially experience worsening of symptoms but over time, symptoms will improve. Beta-blockers work by affecting the response to some nerve impulses in certain parts of the body. As a result, they decrease the heart's need for blood and oxygen by reducing its workload. They also help the heart to beat more regularly:

- Ask your doctor if you should check your pulse before and after taking your beta-blocker. Sometimes, these drugs can slow heart rate too much, creating circulation problems.
- Never stop taking beta-blockers without first checking with your doctor. Stopping beta-blockers suddenly can lead to serious medical problems.

- If you have trouble getting to sleep while taking beta-blockers, take them earlier in the evening (at least two hours before bedtime).
- If you have asthma, make sure your physician is aware of it because beta-blockers may make your asthma worse.
- Report these side effects: Fatigue, difficulty concentrating, insomnia, nightmares, dizziness, slow heart rate (less than 50 beats per minute), wheezing, cold hands and feet.

7.4 Diuretics

Diuretics get rid of water and salt from the body. They prevent or reduce swelling, shortness of breath, and bloating. Some diuretics may also get rid of potassium from your body. You may need to take potassium pills while on diuretics. Take this medication with meals to avoid stomach upset. Take the last dose before 4:00 p.m. to avoid getting up at night to pass water. Sometimes two diuretics may be used to get better relief of symptoms. When you start this medication, you will notice an increase in the amount of water you pass within one day. Some side effects you might experience are:

- Weakness, dizziness;
- Muscle cramps; and
- Nausea, dry mouth, and increased thirst.

7.5 Digoxin

This medication increases the strength of the pumping action of your heart. You should wait two hours after taking antacids or fibre supplements before taking digoxin. You will not feel different immediately after taking this medication, but it is important that you continue to take it. Over time, digoxin should improve your symptoms. Some side effects you might experience are:

- Nausea, vomiting, diarrhea;
- Major loss of appetite, weakness; and
- Blurred vision, confusion.

If these occur contact your doctor immediately. It is important that you do not stop taking any medication without advice from your doctor.

7.6 Hydralazine and Nitrates

Hydralazine widens blood vessels, easing blood flow. Side effects may include headaches, rapid heartbeat, and joint pain. Nitrates are used mostly for chest pain, but may also help diminish heart failure symptoms. They relax smooth muscle and widen blood vessels. They act to lower primarily systolic blood pressure. Side effects may include headaches.

8. CAN A PERSON LIVE WITH HEART FAILURE?

Heart failure is one of the most serious symptoms of heart disease. About two-thirds of all patients die within 5 years of diagnosis. However, some live beyond 5 years, even into old age. The outlook for an individual patient depends on the patient's age, severity of heart failure, overall health, and a number of other factors. As heart failure progresses, the effects can become quite severe, and patients often lose the ability to perform even modest physical activity. Eventually, the heart's reduced pumping capacity may interfere with routine functions, and patients may become unable to care for themselves. The loss in functional ability can occur quickly if heart attacks or the worsening of other conditions that affect heart failure, such as diabetes and coronary heart disease, further weakens the heart. Heart failure patients also have an increased risk of sudden death or cardiac arrest, caused by an irregular heartbeat. To improve the chances of surviving with heart failure, patients must take care of themselves. Patients must:

- ❑ See their physician regularly;
- ❑ Closely follow all of their physician's instructions;
- ❑ Take any medication according to instructions; and
- ❑ Immediately inform their physician of any significant change in their condition, such as an intensified shortness of breath or swollen feet.

Patients with heart failure also should:

- ❑ Control their weight;
- ❑ Watch what they eat;
- ❑ Not smoke cigarettes or use other tobacco products; and
- ❑ Abstain from or strictly limit alcohol consumption.

Even with the best care, heart failure can worsen, but patients who don't take care of them are almost writing themselves a prescription for poor health. The best defense against heart failure is the prevention of heart disease. Almost all of the major coronary risk factors can be controlled or eliminated: smoking, high cholesterol, high blood pressure, diabetes and obesity.

9. WHAT IS THE OUTLOOK FOR HEART FAILURE?

Within the past decade, knowledge of heart failure has improved dramatically but clearly, much more remains to be learned. The National Heart, Lung, and Blood Institute (NHLBI) supports numerous research projects aimed at building on what is already known about heart failure and at uncovering new knowledge about its process, diagnosis, and treatment. NHLBI research priorities for heart failure include:

- ❑ Learning more about basic cellular changes that lead to heart failure;
- ❑ Developing tests to detect the earliest signs of heart failure;
- ❑ Identifying factors that cause heart failure to worsen;
- ❑ Determining how heart failure can be reversed once it starts;
- ❑ Understanding better the heart's ability to compensate for lost pumping ability; and
- ❑ Developing new therapies, especially those based on early signs of heart failure.

10. MAKING THE MOST OF YOUR VISIT TO THE DOCTOR

Contact your doctor, if any of the following occurs:

- ❑ Increased shortness of breath;
- ❑ Weight gain of more than 2 pounds (1 kg) over 2 days, or 5 pounds (3 kg) in a single week;
- ❑ Nausea or vomiting;
- ❑ Bloating or feeling "full" all the time;
- ❑ Cough or cold symptoms that last for 2 weeks or more;
- ❑ Extreme tiredness;
- ❑ Increased swelling of the feet or legs; and
- ❑ Increased urination at night.

Don't hesitate to ask questions to clarify points. Also, ask your doctor to rephrase a reply you cannot understand. Briefly describe your symptoms; even those you feel may not be important. You may want to keep a list so you will remember them—

- ❑ Tell the doctor all of the medications you take—including over-the-counter drugs—and any problems you may be having with them.
- ❑ Be sure you understand all of the doctor's instructions—especially for medications. Know what drug to take when, how often, and in what amount.
- ❑ Find out what side effects are possible from any drug the doctor prescribes for you.
- ❑ Ask the meaning of any medical term you don't understand.
- ❑ If, after your appointment, you still have questions or are uncertain about your treatment, call the doctor's office to get the information you need.
- ❑ With your doctor's permission, try to be as physically active as you can on a regular basis. Ask about enrolling in a cardiac rehabilitation clinic that has a structured and supervised exercise program. Avoid being active right after meals or when it's very hot or humid.

7

Restore Fitness Early: Secondary Prevention in Case of Fracture

R.L. MITTAL*

(I) GENERAL CONSIDERATIONS

At the outset, it may be pointed out that it would be more appropriate to prevent the occurrence of fracture wherever possible. However, once the fracture has occurred prompt detection, treatment and rehabilitation are essential to prevent pain, deformity, disability and death. This is called secondary prevention. This secondary prevention of complications is as important as primary prevention of the occurrence of fracture.

A fracture/dislocation is said to be open when there is an external wound with communication between the fracture and the outside air. Sometimes the wound is small and away from fracture site and the communication with outside air may be devious. On other occasions, there may be a wound directly opposite the fracture site but without communicating

* M.S., F.A.M.S., F.I.C.S., F.A.I.S., Formerly Professor & Head, Department of Orthopaedics, and Principal, Govt. Medical College/Rajindra Hospital, Patiala. Presently, Consultant, Mittal Orthopaedic Centre, 97, New Lal Bagh Colony, Patiala.

with the fracture. So the essential feature for diagnosing an open fracture is its communication with exterior and the presence of an outside wound may often be misleading. The real test of open fracture in doubtful cases is that dark venous blood exudes from the wound which increases on pressing and minute fat droplets can be seen in this blood. An open fracture may be primary, when wound occurs at the time of fracture, and this may be from within caused by fracture fragments or caused by external violence. It may be secondary, when closed fracture has been converted into open by sloughing of soft tissues over it or by a surgical procedure.

An open fracture caused by external violence is always contaminated with bacteria, which occurs at the time of injury persisting till the organisms begin to grow and invade the tissues and the wound becomes actually infected. As regards the time period, it is directly proportional to the amount of outside contamination. Roughly speaking, a fracture is considered only contaminated during the first 6 hours, potentially infected during 6-12 hours and infected after 12 hours. However, in heavily contaminated fractures from outside, the fracture may become infected even earlier and conversely in comparatively clean wounds, infection may be delayed for 24 hours or so. Not only contamination, but tissue damage/devitalisation play an important role for accelerating or decelerating the infective process. The more the damage to tissues the earlier and severer may be the infection.

(II) GENERAL MANAGEMENT

In these days of high speed, life threatening trauma with multiple injuries has become increasingly common and therefore treatment of an open fracture should start at the site of accident before patient is transported to a hospital and receives definitive treatment there.

(A) An Accident Side

It will depend upon; (a) type of injury; (b) locality of accident, and (c) facilities available. If the patient is not severely injured, distance from hospital is short and good transport facilities are available, no special treatment is necessary except first aid to fracture and a clean dressing. Even otherwise, in an open fracture transport to a hospital at the earliest is very important. Importance of first aid to fracture can not be over emphasised and what was true about first aid two centuries ago, holds true even today.

If the patient is seriously injured, it is important that certain measures are taken at the site of accident to maintain airway, prevent shock and prevent further injury, because in a highway accident patient can have multiple injuries to limbs, trunk and head.

A severely injured patient should be moved only after essential life and limb saving measures. Mishandling causes pain, increases shock and further injury to tissues and increase contamination. If the patient is bleeding considerably, it must be stopped by a pressure bandage or, if required, by tourniquet and noting the time of its application.

An open wound should be covered with a clean dressing at the earliest, which not only prevents bleeding but also from further contamination. If sterile dressing is not available, a clean laundered handkerchief will also do the job. The limb should be straightened and simple first aid splint given. Some antibiotic powder can also be used locally, if there is likelihood of delay in definitive treatment.

Efforts should be made to keep the patient warm and dry and nothing should be given by mouth anticipating the requirement of anaesthesia for definitive treatment. On the other hand, injury leads to cessation of peristalsis and hence if the stomach is full at the time of injury, stomach wash may be required. Besides all this an injection of non-narcotic analgesic will reduce pain and thereby shock. If a trained person is available, a broad spectrum antibiotic can also be started which would delay the onset of infection to some extent especially where the definitive treatment is likely to be delayed.

(B) Treatment in the Hospital or Definitive Treatment

"The primary objective in the management of an open fracture is union with prevention or eradication of wound sepsis." The basic principle here again is preservation of life first and for that it is important to see that an adequate airway is there, bleeding is controlled and shock is treated if present. After that a thorough examination of the patient as a whole is carried out in order to assess the extent of injury and to establish the priorities of treatment in case of multiple injuries. Prognosis in open fracture will depend upon the extent of injury. GUSTILLO and ANDERSON type I and II have a favourable prognosis while type III-A, B and C have unfavourable prognosis in descending order. In general, a more extensive damage to the soft tissue denotes an unfavourable prognosis.

If the splinting and dressing have not been done already, this should be done. Antibiotics should be started immediately. After that patient is sent for X-ray examination without any delay and this facility should be available nearest to the emergency room.

(C) Prophylactic Role of A.T.S. and A.G.G.S.

Prophylactic use of A.T.S. is only indicated occasionally in a grossly contaminated wound in an agricultural terrain. Use of prophylactic A.G.G.S. is not indicated. However, active immunisation with tetanus toxoid, in non-immunised and a booster dose in immunised, should always be undertaken. The best prophylaxis against these infections is proper wound management.

(III) TREATMENT OF THE WOUND AND FRACTURE

The aim of treatment is to convert open fracture to a closed one as early as possible with the least risk to the patient. Delay would mean inevitable infection. A thorough debridement of wound is done which means excision of skin margins, dead and devitalised soft tissue, foreign bodies and loose small bits of bone. Sir ALEXANDER FLEMING said, "The greatest of all antiseptics is living tissue." It is only through the intact blood supply of living tissues that the body defences can operate and fight the impending infection and then deliver the raw material of repair to the injured area. Dead and devitalised tissue being without blood supply are not able to have protective influence and rather provide ideal culture medium for organisms including anaerobic ones and infection gets established.

Treatment of the wound should start with cleansing of whole limb by washing, shaving and painting with antiseptic preparation. Cetavlon or Betadine is a good agent for preliminary cleansing. After that it is cleaned with tincture iodine and spirit. Cleansing should be away from the wound and dirty washings should not get into the wound. Limb should be draped as for a clean surgery. Tourniquet should not usually be used as it interferes with the ability to differentiate dead from living tissue and to attain complete haemostasis. However, when excessive bleeding is there or in cases requiring intricate reconstruction, tourniquet can be used. The entire wound should be flushed with adequate saline solution.

Skin

The skin wound should be enlarged as required and edges should be excised till a healthy bleeding edge is obtained. In cases where a large area of skin is lifted from subcutaneous tissue and devitalised, it should be replaced after thorough toilet. In such cases a variable area is likely to survive and after 1-2 weeks the dead skin can be removed and replaced by split skin grafts. Sometimes there is only superficial crushing of skin and deeper layers survive. Skin wound should be closed only if it can be done without undue tension, but every effort should be made to cover an exposed bone. It is not always easy to decide whether to close the wound primarily or not. In general, if the time elapsed is short and reasonable, the soft tissue damage is not much, a complete debridement has been done and there is no undue tension, the wound should be closed primarily. Large wounds, after thorough debridement can be loosely closed. All others should be left open for secondary closure. Whenever in doubt, it is always safe to leave the wound open.

Division of Fascia

Wound should be extended proximally and distally so that all injured deeper tissues can be exposed easily without undue traction. All pockets, intermuscular spaces should be opened and blood clots evacuated so that post-traumatic oedema of muscles does not result in ischaemia and necrosis.

Crushed Muscles

Extent of muscle damage can be assessed by four "Cs"—Colour, consistency, capacity to bleed and contractility of which colour is the least important. A living muscle is shiny, pinkish, elastic to feel, bleeds and contracts on stimulation while a dead muscle is dull, dark brownish, firm, does not bleed or contract. All dead and devitalised muscle tissue must be ruthlessly excised till bleeding muscle tissue is there, so as to avoid infection especially by anaerobic organisms of tetanus and gas gangrene.

Gunshot Wounds

Few gunshot wounds are alike and therefore the same practice can not apply to all (JOHN HUNTER, 1761). The extent of damage will depend upon velocity, size, shape of the shot and resistance encountered. Impact with bone causes wide spread destruction of soft tissues. All these wounds are always contaminated by foreign matter and hence potentially infected. All these wounds require thorough debridement. If entrance and exit wounds are there, both need excision. They should never be closed primarily. Local antibiotic can be put in and they should be loft open.

Removal of Foreign Bodies

Pieces of clothing, wood, glass, dirt and in gunshot injuries fragments of bullet, shell, etc. should be removed. However, where small pellets of shotgun are scattered over a wide area in deeper tissues, they should be left in, as they do not cause much damage. In some cases, of missile injuries large metallic fragments are scattered diffusely and it is not possible to remove all of them and only easily accessible ones should be removed. In general, bullets introduce bacteria in the depth of the wound and behind it there is suction effect leading to sucking in of infected piece of clothing or skin tag. So they need removal whenever possible, especially if some reconstruction with implant is contemplated.

Fragments

Small detached and contaminated pieces of bone should be removed; but large fragments, even if detached, completely, from soft tissues, must be retained in order to prevent gap, non-union and shortening.

Primary Fixation of Fracture

No hard and fast rule can be made about it, but there is no doubt that any internal fixation device will result in more bone necrosis and chances of infection, with plating more so than with I.M. nailing. However, in selected problematic cases, where stabilisation of fracture will offer an advantage in proper wound management or preventing complications, it should be done. This is particularly so when a major vascular injury has been repaired. Intramedullary fixation would be better than plating in such cases. In unstable fractures of tibia, a two pin transfixation with plaster cast is a good method. With the renewed interest and popularity of external fixators, it is worthwhile and extremely gratifying to use external fixation in many of these problem open fractures. It avoids all the complications of internal fixation achieving at the same time the objective of stabilisation of fracture.

Cut Nerves and Tendons

Primary repair of cut nerves should not be done. However ends should be identified and brought nearer with a single black silk stitch for Identification at the time of secondary repair. As regards repair of tendons, flexor tendons in the hand are not repaired primarily. Tendons at the wrist, back of hand, ankle, elbow and knee can be repaired if circumstances permit. In cases of all cut tendons and nerves, internal fixation of fracture will simplify later management of these injuries.

Skin Wound

Primary Closure

Skin protects the deeper soft tissues and bone from infection. Therefore, whenever possible, skin wound should be closed even by giving releasing incision, but there should be no undue tension. Stitching under tension will lead to breaking down and also necrosis of more adjacent skin causing a bigger wound.

Delayed Primary Closure

After waiting for 4-5 days for oedema to subside and if there are no signs of infection, it would be possible to stitch the wound in moderate injuries. The advantage of this is that elasticity of skin is still there and edges have not retracted. But if infection occurs, secondary closure after 10 days will be required. Skin edges may have to be undermined and relaxing incisions may also be required, before closure without tension.

Skin Grafting

When primary or delayed suture is not possible raw area can be covered with split skin grafts to provide a primary dressing even on the bare bone after decorticating it. This will prevent infection. Later on depending upon the requirement of patients, pedicle grafts, free vascularised microsurgical grafts myocutaneous flaps, etc. can be used.

Suction Drainage

This can be used only if complete skin closure has been achieved and is useful in extensive soft tissue damage with inevitable, haematoma in the post-operative period.

Immobilisation in POP

In open fractures, as the fractured fragments are visible, so the fracture should be reduced whenever possible and the fragments held in position before the wound is closed. The limb is then immobilised in plaster cast, which not only immobilises the fracture, but is also an important measure for allowing the soft tissues to heal better and thus avoid infection. The limb is then elevated for the swelling to subside.

Traction

Quite often, open fracture may have to be treated by skin or skeletal traction, e.g. when the patient has other serious injuries and patient is unfit for anaesthesia or in cases of unstable fractures. It is important to maintain good alignment of fracture during the waiting period in the hope that fracture union will occur in good position.

(IV) POST-OPERATIVE MANAGEMENT

This includes elevation of the part, antibiotics, supportive treatment, watching the patient for any evidence of infection and treating it, if it is there. If the wound has been closed, it should not be disturbed till about the 10th day, when stitches can be removed by cutting a window in plaster and dressing applied again. Position of the fracture should also be checked by X-ray after 3 weeks. In the cases, where wound has been left open, they should be closed after 4-5 days by delayed primary closure.

Evidence of infection will be indicated by increased pain, rise in pulse rate, fever and leukocytosis. In such cases, window is made in plaster to inspect the wound which will be oedematous and discharging. Stitches are removed and drained. Pus should be cultured and sensitivity tested and patient is put on appropriate antibiotics.

Gas Gangrene

Whenever infection is suspected it is extremely important to find out whether it is pyogenic or due to gas gangrene. In latter, there is excruciating pain, patient is very ill looking and there is disproportionate rise in pulse rate to increase in temperature. The skin around the wound is tense, copper coloured with exudation of thin typical foul smelling discharge which increases on pressure. The smell is typical and once recognised it is never forgotten. There are gas bubbles in this discharge and gas crepitus in the soft tissues. Smear from the discharge shows short thick bacilli in large numbers. Skiagram also shows, later on, evidence of gas. It should be remembered that sometimes air may be entrapped in the dead spaces in the tissues as in surgical emphysema. This has to be differentiated from the gas gangrene, because one is absolutely innocuous and other one is mostly fatal. Gas gangrene is of 3 degrees

(1) degree—only localised around the wounds,
(2) degree—localised to one muscle or one group of muscles, and
(3) degree—extensive infection.

Early diagnosis is very important for saving the life and limb of the patient and treatment is surgical. All stitches are removed and wound extended widely to remove the dead muscles and drained freely. If it is extensive involving all fascial planes, limb is amputated. Anti-gas gangrene serum is given (50,000 units) after careful sensitivity test. Penicillin is still the best antibiotic and tetracyclines can also be added. Hyperbaric oxygen is also useful which acts by stopping toxin production and improving the oxygenation of tissues.

Tetanus Infection

This also is a serious infection. The incubation is 10-90 days and more the incubation period, the better is the prognosis. Infection may be of 3 degrees—

(1) degree—only localised rigidity,
(2) degree—generalised rigidity, and
(3) generalised rigidity and recurrent reflex spasms. Earlier the spasm develop, poorer is the prognosis.

Prophylactic ATS is only very rarely indicated. However, active immunisation should be carried out. There are 4 principles of management in preventing tetanus—

(a) Adequate wound debridement, which is the best prophylax is.
(b) Systemic antibiotics—penicillin should be started at the earliest.
(c) ATS—only occasionally.
(d) Active immunisation—always.

In the treatment of an established case wound should be thoroughly explored, excised and dressed open. Full dose of penicillin should be given. ATS in the dose of 1-2 lac units should be given after sensitivity test. If the patient is sensitive to horse serum, human ATS is given in the dose of 20,000 to 40,000 units. Besides of course sedatives are given for control of spasms.

(V) PYOGENIC INFECTED WOUNDS

Some of the patients who have been treated by the above measures may get infected or they may come late. It may be mild or severe and usually of mixed organisms. Problems in these cases are two-fold:

(1) Problem of management of fracture.
(2) Problem of managing infection.

Various measures required will vary from patient to patient. If there is shock, supportive treatment will be necessary along with blood transfusion, antibiotics and adequate open drainage. It is important to maintain a satisfactory position of the fragments by plaster immobilisation with a good window or skin/skeletal traction and doing dressings without disturbing the fracture. External fixation very often serves as a good method of managing the wound as well as the fracture. If an internal fixation has been used, it is not disturbed at this stage. With this treatment, infection may heal and fracture may unite quite often. If the fracture does not unite but infection heals, this will have to be treated like other non-unions.

(VI) OLD INFECTED OPEN FRACTURES

Quite often infection does not heal and osteomyelitis develops. It differs from ordinary haematogenous osteomyelitis in that the infection is limited near the fracture site only. The management will differ from case to case. They may come with fracture uniting or undergoing non-union. Others may be with internal fixation with or without union. Still others may be with foreign bodies. If the fracture is uniting, it is imperative to wait till the involucrum is strong and then we can perform sequestrectomy and/or removal of implant. If there is no progress of union after waiting adequately, sequestrectomy and or removal of implant has to be carried out and the non union shall have to be dealt with later on when the infection has healed. If this non-union is with gap, this will require its own treatment by various methods available. Sometimes unusual foreign bodies may be the cause of discharging sinus and not osteomyelitis and the fracture has healed. Scrapping and removal of foreign body will be required in such cases after doing sinogram with methylene blue.

(VII) REPLACENET OF UNSTABLE SCARS

In open fractures, the fracture may heal with an unstable, repeatedly breaking down scar. At other times, fractures have not healed with non-union with or without gap or malunions. These scars will have to be replaced by full thickness skin either pedicle grafts, or free vascularised grafts. This will be necessary for carrying out necessary reconstruction, as one can have good healing only if healthy skin is available over the reconstructed area.

(VIII) PROPHYLACTIC BONE GRAFTING

Autogenous cancellous bone grafting should be strongly considered for open fractures that are not progressing to union roentgenographically by 12 weeks.

Recently bone graft substitutes been used in place of autogenous graft. Collagraft (60% Hydroxyapatite and 40% tricalcium phosphate, ciramic and fibriliar). When mixed with autogenous bone marrow, acts as autogenous graft. So this can be used where large amount of cancellous graft is required.

(IX) AMPUTATION

Occasionally, for badly crushed limbs with eurovascular compromise, amputation may have to be done. The recent advances in the management of open fracture has permitted the development of techniques that result in salvageable but non-functional limbs. In such conditions patient is not affected only physically but also psychologically, financially and socially. Sometimes inevitable amputations are delayed too long.

Several attempts have been made for better election of injury pattern that would be treated by early amputation. Mangled extremity severity score (MESS) formulated by HELFET DL *et al* in 1990, when combined with clinical experience of the surgeon is a very good guide in this aspect.

It is based on '4' group systems—

(1) Skeletal and Soft Tissue Injuries
(2) Shock
(3) Tschaemia
(4) Age

MESS of 7-12 usually require amputation while between 3-6 results in viable limbs.

However, judgement of an experienced surgeon is very important depending upon case to case for taking a final decision about amputation.

Mangled Extremity Severity Score

Type Characteristics	*Injuries*	*Points*
1. Skeletal/soft tissue group		
(a) Low energy	Stab wound, closed fracture, small calibre gun shot	1
(b) Medium energy	Open/multiple level fractures dislocation massive crush injury	2
(c) High energy	Close range, high velocity gunshots	3
(d) Massive Crush	Logging, railroad, oil rig accidents	4
2. Shock group		
(a) Normotensive haemodynamics	BP stable in field and in operation room (OR)	0
(b) Transiently hypotensive	BP unstable in field but responsive to I/V fluids	1
(c) Prolonged hypotensive	Systolic BP less than 90 mm of Hg. in field but responsive to I/V fluids in OR only	2

3. Ischaemia group		
(a) None	A pulsatile limb without sign of ischaemia	0
(b) Mild	Diminished pulses without sign of ischaemia	1
(c) Moderate	No pulse by Doppler, sluggish capillary refill paraesthesia, diminished motor activity	2
(d) Advanced	Pulses, cool, paralysed and numb without capillary refill than 50 yrs.	3
4. Age group		
(a) Less than 30 yrs.		0
(b) More than 30 yrs. less		1
(c) More than 50 yrs.		2

(X) REHABILITATION

Rehabilitation of patient and extremity should begin immediately depending upon the fracture and soft tissues stability. Physical therapy with active and active assisted exercises for joint mobilisation should start as soon as soft issue healing permits. Neurologic deficits if any should be related by splinting of joints in functional position to avoid contractures. Weight bearing should be monitored closely. Joint Movements and strengthening exercise should also be continued. Finally, the patient should be instructed as to his responsibility for maximum functional return of the limb. Vocational rehabilitation should be initiated early to provide a productive return to society.

Open fracture, if managed with care at the earliest, should give satisfying results, on the other hand, delay and carelessness in treatment will lead to disastrous complications, which can even be life threatening.

8

Your Fitness, Your Health: You are the Custodian

B.K. Chopra* and Vishal Chopra**

"Be merry and happy" should be the motto of every one as you will not pass through this world again. Have you ever realized that you are the most lucky person as God Almighty has given you human body which is priceless? Even if the whole world is on one side, one cannot purchase a natural little finger what to talk of the whole body.

Nature has gifted you with special sense organs, i.e. eyes to see natural beauty, ears to hear and enjoy music, tongue to enjoy taste of good food, nose to enjoy good smell and fragrance. It is your responsibility to take care of your body. You are the custodian of your own health and your own body. The old proverb "When wealth is lost, nothing is lost, When health is lost, something is lost, When character is lost everything is lost" needs modification "When health and/or character are lost, everything is lost.

* (Ex) Professor and Head, Department of Medicines, Government Medical College, Patiala.

** Pulmonologist.

WHAT IS HEALTH?

It is difficult to define health. It is more of your mental attitude. Health is not merely an absence of disease.

Health is defined as:

(i) Physical Health

The presence or absence of disease.

(ii) Mental Health

"A sound mind in a sound body."

(iii) Social Health

That means you are a good human being with good human values.

(iv) Spiritual Health

Provides you inner strength.

The medical science has made tremendous progress in the last 3 decades in the field of diagnosis and treatment. The newer machines that are too costly have come in the market like CT scans, MRI scans, endoscopies, Angiographies and so on. The latest treatments like laser, heart surgery, brain surgery are beyond the reach of common man. So one must realize that medical treatment in the modern era is too costly a commodity. God forbid, if you fall ill with a serious illness, the cost of the treatment can ruin all your earnings. Many a time, the treatment overall in most of the cases will only give you limited help.

A very important fact to realize is that inspite of the latest advances in the field of medicine, availability of specialist/super specialist care, we have not achieved the goal for good health. The goal of health for all is a distant dream. Still, millions of people are suffering from diseases like high blood pressure, diabetes, heart attacks, strokes, i.e. paralysis, cancer, AIDS and STDs (Sexually transmitted diseases), crippling deformities due to automobile accidents.

Inspite of the lack of medical facilities, because of the active life, the people in old times were healthier and physically stronger. If we ponder the simple reason of poor health in modern times is the sedentary lifestyle, lazy habits, lack of physical activity, faulty food habits, overuse of the automobiles and over and above mental stress of modern life.

PARAMETERS OF HEALTH

The parameters of health are many like height, weight, blood pressure, heart rate, pulse rate, respiratory rate and biochemical parameters like blood sugar level, blood urea level for kidney assessment, blood cholesterol for body fats, blood uric acid levels for joint pains, bilirubin level for liver and so on. There are lot of variations of these parameters and it is just not possible to draw a strict line between normal and abnormal. If you start investigating your body intricately with all the tests available at your disposal, you are bound to detect some abnormality some where and you will be labeled a sick person which in fact you may not be. Simple criteria of good health are if you can perform your day-to-day activities without any discomfort and infirmity, can digest food, have good appetite, comfortable sleep, proper response to nature's call regularly, feel reasonably, fit mentally, physically and are not having any symptoms, you are a healthy person.

Once you get some signal that indicates some kind of disturbance, you may consult your doctor. Health is a relative feeling. If you meet people around you who are very sick and disabled you will feel comparatively healthy even if you are a little sick and you will feel thankful to nature.

You are most lucky person if you are having no disease at all. You are still lucky if the disease you are suffering from does not interfere with daily activities. You will feel miserable if you are bedridden and you cannot perform daily routine activities.

HOW TO KEEP GOOD HEALTH

The road to good health is a long journey. It starts at birth, even earlier when one is in the womb of one's mother when she takes care of your health by a good prenatal care, i.e. good lifestyle, walks, proper vaccination and a positive healthy mind. The health of an individual is determined by genetic and environmental factors. Genetic predisposition is a tendency that you inherit from your parents and is not under your control. However, the environmental influences which cause so many acquired diseases, can be controlled or modified.

The old dictum "Prevention is better than cure", "A stitch in time saves nine." Prevention is still the cheapest method to preserve good health.

Health is a matter of lifestyle and to have good health you should have good and healthy lifestyle right from childhood when you should do good physical activity, play games, have good nutritious diet rich in proteins, vitamins, minerals like milk, curd, cheese, fruits, green vegetables, eggs, meat, etc., avoid taking junk food, inculcate discipline and good habits which make you a good human being with good human values, a kind sympathetic, sincere, hard working citizen and overall a smart, good looking young man with healthy reddish complexion so that society appreciates you and recognizes you. **"Healthy mother, healthy father, healthy children, healthy youth and a healthy nation."**

The pivot of most of the diseases like high blood pressure, sugar (diabetes), heart diseases, paralysis, stomach ulcers, AIDS and even cancer is stress of modern life, faulty food habits and an unhealthy lifestyle. Be ambitious but not over ambitious. Work in the right direction so that you can achieve the goal, shed anxiety and depression, avoid stress, have positive thinking, think good of others. Even if you have stress, take it in a positive way since it conditions your mind and body to solve the problem.

"All leisure, no stress, road to death."
"Smile, that way the world looks better."
" Mind in its own way and in itself can make heaven of hell and a hell of heaven."
"Depression is a slow poison. Be careful lest you ingest it."

To keep physically fit, adopt some simple principles:

1. Have an active daily routine. Use your legs more than automobile. Daily morning walk for 1/2-1 hr with light body exercises, may be even yoga exercises should be made a daily routine.

2. *Diet*: Sedentary workers (desk workers): do not overeat, eat less food, nutritious food rich in vitamins, minerals, green leafy vegetables, fruit, eggs, meat, juice. Hard working persons and manual labourers need more diet. Young growing children also need more diet and a rich protein diet. Overeating, excess fat intake leads to diet-related diseases like high blood pressure, high blood cholesterol which causes heart attacks and paralysis, high blood sugar, i.e. diabetes, arthritis like gout. One should avoid overeating. **"Eat to live and not live to eat."** No man has died of hunger but a man can die of overeating. One should take less food and seasonal items.

Of course, food requirements vary from person to person depending on the nature of his job. One should not adopt defective food habits. In growing age upto 20 years one can take four basic meals, from 20-30 yrs. three basic meals, from 30-40 years two main meals with fruits and vegetables, after 40 years one main meal with fruits, vegetables, juice, snacks, etc.

3. Regular fast one day in a week is certainly good. But fast should be fast in true sense. One may take fruit, juice, etc. on the day of fast. Fasting for 2-3 continuous days after a gap of few months will certainly improve your health and body parameters like blood sugar, blood cholesterol and will keep your body weight under control.

4. *Personal hygiene and clothes*: Have daily bath, in summer 2-3 times only regular nail cutting, hair cutting. Brush your teeth in morning and night and after each meal. Prefer cotton clothes, avoid synthetic clothes as these cause skin diseases.

5. Sex Education so that you do not succumb to AIDS and STDS.

6. *Automobile Drive at safe speed*: **"Safety saves."** Use of mobile phones, high speed driving under tension and under the effect of drugs, i.e. addiction can cause accidents and make you invalid and crippled.

7 *Regular medical check-up*: After the age of 40, you should undergo regular medical check-up like blood pressure, heart examination, blood sugar (for diabetes) blood urea (for kidney assessment), blood cholesterol, lipid profile for the risk of heart attacks and strokes (paralysis), ECG for heart, X-ray chest for lungs, may be even an ultra sound of the abdomen.

8. Try to keep carefree life and have sound sleep but not by medicines.

9. Try to keep mental peace, relaxed mind, avoid anger, don't keep anxiety or feeling of frustration. Try to gain spiritual strength.

10. Keep your weight under control, avoid overeating and resort to regular walk and exercise. Overweight causes heart attacks, diabetes, strokes, arthritis and high blood pressure.

11. To avoid day-to-day infection observe following precautions:

(a) Clean/wash your hands and spoon before eating food and drinking water.
(b) Avoid eating stored food, ready made food, left out food, fast food. Avoid too spiced, fried food which causes stomach cancer.
(c) Prefer hot drinks. Drink purified/chlorinated, boiled and then cooled/aquafiltered water. Cold drinks should be taken with precaution. Milk products like ice cream and sweets left over for sometime should be avoided.
(d) Avoid congested places or close contact with patients suffering from flue, chronic cough, tuberculosis and infectious illnesses.
(e) Avoid dust, smoke and living in congested cites. They can produce nasal allergies, skin diseases and Asthma. (See Appendix III: 'Nasal Allergies' to know more about this common problem).

12. Proper vaccination as advised by your doctor prevents many infectious diseases.

13. *Addiction*: **Stay away from addiction.**

A healthy lifestyle is a matter of habit and daily routine which should start with the first breath in the morning after a fresh, sound and comfortable sleep at night without mental tension.

The first thing should be a morning walk for half to one hour with simple exercises followed by daily bath, care of body parts like teeth, nails, hair and skin then prayer for a while if you believe in the laws of nature. Read newspaper then have a nutritious breakfast consisting of milk, fruit, bread, egg, little cheese, curd and may be even some fruit, cornflakes and porridge. Avoid eating in between the meals but you can have a cup of tea/milk, a banana/apple/orange, few biscuits or green vegetables. Lunch should be light consisting of 1-2 chappatis, curd, seasonal vegetables and a fruit. In between lunch and dinner one can have a snack/ sandwich, a cup of milk or a fruit. One can also have lemonade or *lassi*. One should go for an evening walk. Dinner should be lighter than lunch. A stroll for about 15-20 minutes will help one in digesting the food. The principles of diet are not so rigid. One can enjoy an ice-cream, a cold drink, other fried things and non-vegeterian items but do not take liberties. The best one can do is that once overeating has been done one should skip the next meal. The old dictums "An apple a day keeps the doctor away" or "A banana a day keeps the heart attacks away" still hold true. One should try to take 5-10 minutes nap after breakfast called a "luxury nap", about half an hour nap after lunch called "siesta." It is well said: "A siesta a day keeps the heart attacks away." During day-to-day activities one should try to do a lot of walking and use stairs.

Smoking should be avoided. It damages the lungs, causes heart attacks, lung cancer and paralysis. Alcohol should be taken in moderation. Excessive use of alcohol damages the liver, heart and nerves of the body and also causes stomach ulcer. Tobacco chewing also causes mouth cancer.

Avoid anger. Greet people with a smile. Have positive thinking. Do not shout. You will loose good will and reputation and you will increase your own mental tension. People have suffered heart attacks during a fit of emotions and extreme anger. Use soft and pleasant words that cost nothing. Each minute is a lost minute. Utilize it properly. Be honest and upright, do not deceive and do not tell a lie, do not steel. Spread message of good will, love and affection. Spread fragrance around you. Serve the society in the most humble way. Serve the elderly, serve your parents, help the poor, needy and down-trodden.

All this what I have mentioned above appears a religious discourse. But rest assure, with all the good deeds you will emerge a wonderful human being with good mental health and in turn good physical health. You will love people and people in turn will love you and then you will enjoy the taste of these things.

So the message is that if each one of us adopts a healthy physical, mental, social and spiritual lifestyle the world will become a heaven to live in.

CONCLUSION

Health is a matter of lifestyle and attitude. Health means happiness. Good physical activity, healthy food habits, relaxed mind, simple good habits and overall and above positive thinking are the keys to good health.

9

Modern Lifestyle and Depression: A Healthy Mind Assures a Healthy and Fit Body

RAJEEV GUPTA*

A new phenomenon is gradually emerging, death wish has become a common preoccupation in modern life. Common man has started viewing suicide as a way of getting out of tortuous living. He feels that out of various options available to him, suicide is the easiest one. It is indeed a dangerous trend. Those having moderate and severe depression are knocking at the doors of psychiatrists for help. But they constitute a very small fraction of these patients. In a recent study done in the Dayanand Medical College, Ludhiana, 100 suicide attempts were analyzed. A majority of them suffered from depression. Most of them were not taking any treatment for their problem. Illiteracy, ignorance and poverty still loom large on the Indian horizon. When in distress, the common man does not know what to do. At which door he should knock? He feels quite helpless. Administration is indifferent, the family system has lost its

* Psychiatrist at "MANAS"—Psychology, Epilepsy & Deaddiction Center, Tagore Nagar, Near Hero Heart Center, Ludhiana.

bonds and the traditional communities with tribal bonds have disappeared. There is no anchor for majority of the people. Migration from villages to cities, from poor and backward states to industrialized states continues unabated. More and more people are falling a pray to rootlessness that leads to alienation, despair and then depression.

Those who are reporting to psychiatrists and counselors form just the tip of the iceberg, for they form a very small fraction of the affected population. Majority of them, unable to avail of any medical service, continue to suffer. Depressed patients with physical symptoms are going to medical or surgical clinics. They are getting tonics, painkillers, tranquillizers and sedatives. Most of them are getting an inadequate treatment. Doctors call them 'functional cases'. Visit the clinic of a cardiologist, a chest physician, a gastroenterologist or a neurologist in any city, you will find that it is flooded with cases of functional diseases. They are not suffering from any specific physical illness. If you talk to them or enquire about their mental condition, you will find out that more than half of them are suffering from depression.

They fail to express their inner feelings of sadness and sense of hopelessness. They are unable to talk to doctors about their psychological fears. They present with physical symptoms of depression. In a study, I analyzed symptoms of depressive patients in the Psychiatry OPD of Dayanand Medical College, Ludhiana and found more than half of the cases complained of physical symptoms what psychiatrists call 'somatic symptoms'. Physicians and surgeons cannot treat each and every symptom, for an understanding of the psychological basis of patient's complaints is essential to fully diagnose and treat the patient.

Talk to any school teacher, parent or a child psychiatrist, you will discover that more and more children and adolescents are suffering from depression. They present with physical, psychological and behavioural problems. Some of them feel so low that they even express the idea of ending their lives. Pressure from all the aspects are increasing on them. School and college education is gradually becoming a constant source of stress. Deterioration in the system of education is worrying parents and children. Education is being treated like any other trade. Students are being constantly deprived of quality education. One must admit that today, there is hardly any section of society that has escaped the onslaught of depression. Widening gulf between unending aspirations and diminishing hopes of fulfilment have led to frustration, unhappiness, sadness, rejection and self-dejection among common man. Everyone is striving hard to achieve the impossible. Each one of us wants to emerge victorious. No one is willing to face failure. Each one wants to reach the Mount Everest of his ambitions. Somehow a feeling has come up in the common man that he deserves each and every comfort of life. He loathes tolerating if those luxuries are denied to him. Modern Indian is intolerant and restless. A complete alienation from time tested old traditions and philosophical way of life has added to his frustration, restlessness and depression. Even his religion, heavily loaded with symbols and rituals is unable to give peace and tranquility to his disturbed state of mind.

A recent survey, conducted by a national magazine on the role of status symbols among young executives has revealed that every young man is in a hurry to achieve the best things around him; irrespective of the means he may employ to reach his cherished goal. Ethics have lost their relevance in this journey to progress and prosperity. Veneration has shifted from the gods to the mammon. Narrow outlook has replaced the message of the Gita.

Materialism—a mirage, the Maya has become the badge of modern life. Today in our society at one end of the spectrum most of the people are just striving to survive and at the other end Mercedes-Benz and palatial mansions have become the ultimate parameter of worth and success in life. Under ever-rising stress of breaking people, both from inside and outside, people with limited mental, physical and social resources are being pushed to the wall and feel themselves completely immobilized and handicapped by the fast emerging depression. Today, word "Depression" is no longer confined to the psychiatrist's mind. It is being experienced and can be seen perched on drooping eyes and pale cheeks of most of the people, specially the inhabitants of large towns and thickly populated cities. It is indeed strange that depression, like death, is a greater leveler, for it spares neither the pauper nor the prince. Depression attracts a multidisciplinary approach. In some patients medical psychotherapy, yoga and meditation may be sufficient, but in others one may have to start an adequate treatment. In the following pages, I am giving a brief outline of different modalities used to help depressed people.

MEDICAL TREATMENT

Depressed patients often consult family physicians, medical specialists, psychiatrists or counselors for help. They present with various physical, psychological or behaviour complaints. Studies have shown that 30-40 percent patients attending various health centers in our country do not have any specific physical disease. They only have physical symptoms. Such patients are often made to undergo a series of expensive laboratory tests including ultrasound, EEG, TMT and CT scans, etc. It has been observed that when doctors fail to make a medical diagnosis in such cases, they call them 'functional', meaning thereby that patients are having a psychological problem. As has been pointed out, depression manifests with both physical and psychological symptoms. Stress activates certain specific parts of the nervous system called limbic system, which is connected with many body organs through a wide network of autonomic nerves. An excessive activation of autonomic nervous system can produce symptoms in the chest, heart, abdomen, eyes, mouth, face or limbs and many other parts of the body. One can experience pain, discomfort, weakness, etc. One can feel the beat of the heart or even experience a missing heartbeat. In some cases even the breathing rate may increase. Many patients who are unable to analyze their psychological melodies, attribute these symptoms to a known physical disease. Some patients are so strongly convinced that they suffer from a physical disease; they do not want to entertain the idea that their own emotions are responsible for their physical symptoms. A few of them even undergo surgeries like appendicectomy, cholecystectomy or hysterectomy without any improvement.

In many Western countries, people have been consulting psychiatrists even for their day-to-day problems. They regularly visit them for guidance and counseling. However, in many parts of India, even today visiting a psychiatrist or a counselor is considered a taboo. Many family doctors and physicians hesitate to refer these 'functional' cases to psychiatrists. I have seen even doctors who start treating their own psychological problems or those of their family members without taking help of experts and thus suffer in the long-run. They have a social inhibition of visiting a psychiatrist. However, once these doctors realize the significance and benefits of psychiatric consultation, they get encouraged to refer such cases. Psychiatrists have a medical background with an added advantage of having training in diagnosing and treating psychological problems. Their understanding of such problems is better than that of their other medical- colleagues. They have expertise in handling emotional cases.

ANTI-ANXIETY DRUGS

These are among the most commonly used drugs in medical practice. They reduce anxiety levels and are effective in almost all kind of anxieties, Irrespective of the cause. Common anti-anxiety drugs are chlordiazepoxide, Diazepam, clonazepam, oxazepam and alprazolam. Alprazolam is the most recent drug. It acts very fast and stays in blood for much lesser time than other drugs. It is becoming highly popular among both doctors and patients. I have seen even some child specialists prescribing these drugs to their young patients. These drugs have been widely accepted as anti-stress drugs. Many people take these drugs quite regularly for one reason or another.

They perceive that these drugs help them face problems of life and soothe their nerves. However, such drugs should not be taken without the advice of the doctor, as an excess reliance on them may result in dependence and decrease one's capacity to face routine problems. They cause both physical and psychological dependence. Brain cells get used to the presence of these Drugs. Those who are hooked on to these drugs find it difficult to leave them. If a patient misses even one dose, he gets a craving to take the tablet. Some patients get a feeling of nausea, vomiting, sleep disturbance, Irritability and depression as withdrawal symptoms after missing the drug for a day or two. Others become completely confused. These drugs are to be used only in emergency or in the event of severe problems.

ANTI-DEPRESSANT DRUGS

They form a very important group of drugs for treating depression. Commonly used anti-depressant drugs are imipramine, sertraline, venlafaxine, fluoxetine, paroxetine, fluvoxamine, mianserine and amitriptyline. These drugs should not be taken without medical advice. For one episode of depression one should take an anti-depressant for at least 4-6 months. These drugs have been extensively used throughout the world. Doctors have acquired good experience of using these drugs. In the normal therapeutic dose they do not cause any disabling side effects. Common adverse effects of these drugs are constipation, dryness of mouth, giddiness, fine tremors of hands, etc.

Gradually one gets used to the side effects of these drugs. Some patients of depression make suicidal attempt by taking an overdose of these anti-depressants. This phenomenon is very common in the West. It is advisable to keep these drugs away from the patients, under lock and key. Children should not have access to these drugs. Anti-depressant drugs are far less habit forming than anti-anxiety drugs. They are effective in all types of depression.

PRAYER

Prayer is a total self-surrender to the Ultimate Power or the Divine Will that has created this wonderful world of shifting shadows. It is an expression of gratitude to the Maker by way of thanksgiving for His bounties. He has blessed us with joy and solace in sorrow. If we elevate the self to a higher plane of reality and have the faith in His benevolence and grace, it relieves us from many tensions, which we fail to resolve at our own level. It explains why we kneel down to pray in a moment of crisis or distress and seek this support to gain fortitude and peace. Prayer thus makes us feel mentally secure and strong. A feeling of submission to the Supreme power lightens our burden and sustains us to endure suffering as His test of our faith in the hour of sorrow and pain. It is commonly shared experience that under any threat, our thoughts always go to our mother. She is a symbol of protection and security. Similarly for man 'God' is the source of ultimate protection, security and solace. Prayer would prove a boon to those who remain tense and depressed and suffer the consequent mental pain and confusion. Tension starts telling upon their nerves and affects mental functioning. They lack concentration and hesitate to take decisions or else take wrong decisions. Their negative mental attitude starts coloring every aspect of their life. Unwanted fears and apprehensions build-up in their minds and grip them. They remain in a state of perpetual bewilderment. In my practice, I have found many of my depressed and tense patients, visiting religious places and shrines and performing rituals to come out of their disturbed mental state.

Prayer brings peace look at the faces of those who daily pray. We find an aura of peace and tranquility around them. They have conditioned their minds in such a way that they take tension in their stride and do not fall a prey to depression. They become less apprehensive of future problems, for they leave everything to the Lord. If they ever face a problem, they strongly feel that the Almighty would extend them a helping hand. They always feel that they are being guided by the Divine Will and thus resign themselves to it. A young child playing near his mother always feels secure as long as he can see her or listen to her voice. If he can't see her or can't even listen to her, he becomes upset, feels insecure and starts crying. Those who pray regularly, have faith that they are under the watchful eyes of the Lord. They don't work like thieves; they know He is watching them everywhere. Prayer builds immunity from disease when we pray; we admit our smallness in this vast universe. This feeling of humility provides us strength and courage. Prayer helps us to acquire human virtues and teach us to adopt a model code of conduct. Scientific studies have shown that prayers help improve our resistance against disease and stress. It is thought that our mental status can determine the status of human cells. You may be surprised to know that your emotional status of happiness, sadness, positivity or negativity can decide the immunity status of our body. Cardiologists have seen that those who are very hostile or full of negative emotions are more exposed to the risk of a heart attack.

In fact, men of God remain serene and joyous even in the hour of pain. Swami Rama Krishna suffered from throat cancer but never complained of discomfort or pain. People, who pray daily, have lower incidence of high blood pressure, migraine and other psychosomatic diseases. I have seen many patients who came out of depression by praying alone. There are many instances where regular prayers have helped patients of even cancer to fight the disease successfully.

EXERCISE

Ability to indulge in physical activity is one of the beautiful privileges of life. Natural exercise was a routine with our ancestors, for they were engaged in agriculture, which demanded strenuous physical work. Now most of us are engaged in sedentary professions and remain glued to our chairs for most of the day finding no time to stretch our limbs. We, no longer like walking, which was regarded as a natural human activity, for we prefer to use vehicles to move to places, even to cover short distances. Even in villages, machines are replacing manpower, making people physically slow and less active.

Stress makes muscles tense and causes fatigue of mind and body. During stress, impulses go from the brain to body muscles and result in muscular contraction. Chronic stress leads to chronic muscle tension. Subsequently, people under chronic stress suffer from fatigue. Mental stress may lead to headache, pain in the neck, backache, etc. I know many patients who suffer relapse of backache during acute stress.

It is common to see housewives coming from well-to-do families complaining of lethargy, fatigue, body aches and depression. There is hardly anything they do in their home. The servants do every work. They have a pathologically inactive life. I advise my patients regular exercise to seek relief from mental tension and depression. It has helped hundreds of my patients. A person who walks or takes exercise daily, remains cheerful and happy the whole day. Scientists have concluded that lethargy and depression go hand in hand.

HOW DOES EXERCISE MAKE YOU HAPPY?

Exercise releases a number of chemicals in the body called endorphins, which like morphine, stimulate brain cells. These mentally stimulating chemicals impart a feeling of cheerfulness to the mind. Regular exercise tones up our muscles and keeps the brain alert. It burns away unnecessary calories in the body and saves one from obesity. One looks smart and active and radiates energy; a positive attitude is developed towards life and its problem. Regular exercise is good for diabetics and those who suffer from hypertension. Under the guidance of their specialist, heart patients can also do regular simple exercise.

MEDITATION

Meditation in one or another form has been advocated by all religions and philosophers. Today, human mind has become highly restive. Because of the fast increasing complexities of modern life, there is growing realization across the world to practise meditation in order to come unscathed from the worldly chaos and disharmony. Even regular living tests our coping mechanisms. Basal anxiety levels of the modern man remain always high. He has to keep his mind in a hyperactive state. His mind is constantly loaded with thoughts and ideas. Meditation, in today's world has a great role to play. It cools down our brain cells. All of us know the role of a coolant in our car engine. It does not allow the temperature of the engine to go very high. Those who drove a Fiat car in the past remember how the car had to be stopped after some time and the water had to be repeated put to bring down the temperature. Modern cars have fans in front of the engines that automatically start working the moment the temperature of an engine goes beyond a particular level. They also have high quality coolants.

There are no inbuilt coolants and fans in our brain. Regular meditation plays a very important role to act like a coolant. It helps calm down the excited or hyper excited brain cells. It also helps to clear our brain of unnecessary thoughts and reduces the loaded anxieties. Role of meditation in calming down the autonomic nervous system has been fully established by medical scientists in many research experiments. Experts on meditation claim that it makes our mind relaxed and completely thought-free. One thing is quite certain that those who do regular meditation experience more peaceful moments and remain relaxed compared to those who don't meditate. Meditation helps a person to plunge deep into his mind and equip him with the expertise to drive energy and solace in order to have a smooth sail in this turbulent world.

ANTI-STRESS DIET

All living beings including human organism need a balanced diet. Animals are blessed by the Mother Nature to eat by instinct. No one guides them about the choice of food. They can select their food even during different physical ailments. Many scientists are taking the clue from this animal behaviour to discover new medicines for various medical problems. Man alone has the ability to exercise his choice in food. He can create new foods and diets. He can change his eating habits. In a family of four persons, each may have different likings and eating habits. Running of any vehicle depends upon the quality of fuel. Similarly, balanced diet is needed to maintain a healthy psychophysical individual. It is a common observation that malnutrition leads to physical and mental ailments. The undernourished have poor threshold for stress tolerance. They are more prone to infections and many other physical illnesses. It has been scientifically established that chronic malnutrition leads to low intelligence in children. Fresh fruits and vegetables are anti-stress diets. They contain Antioxidants, which remove free radicals from the human body. Free radicals, products of metabolism in the human body, cause illnesses like high blood pressure, heart ailments and even cancer. Vitamin E has been considered to be an effective anti-oxidant. Studies have shown that natural vitamin E is superior to the synthetic vitamin. A regular intake of Vitamin C reduces stress and thus lemon, amla, imli and oranges rich in vitamin C are beneficial to us.

FOOD ITEMS TO AVOID

Caffeine

It is a brain stimulant. Beverages likes' coffee and tea are rich in caffeine. It is also found in chocolate and cola drinks. Caffeine intake releases a number of chemicals in the brain. It activates brain cells. It releases more energy than is needed at a given time. Once you take caffeine, you consume your future energy also. It is like flogging a fatigue horse to make it run. This is the reason you feel energetic after taking a cup of coffee but after reaching a peak of mental alertness, start feeling low. Caffeine has the tendency to make you dependent. Brain cells get used to certain levels of caffeine in the blood. Regular caffeine intake increases anxiety levels. It makes one more prone to day-to-day stress.

Fats

A diet rich in fats makes you lazy and slow. Fats get easily deposited in the body. Once deposited, they cannot be mobilized easily. Obese people shun physical activity and are prone to overeating and depression. Studies have shown that many depressed patients have high cholesterol level in blood. Inactive people are the easy victim of stress.

Carbohydrates

Diet has to be sufficiently rich in carbohydrates as they provide fuel to the body. Wheat, rice, maize, potatoes are rich in carbohydrates. An individual on low carbohydrate diet will have less body fuel and energy. Brain deprived of regular energy becomes prone to stress. Children particularly expend a lot of energy and need a carbohydrate-rich diet.

Proteins

They make body building blocks. A growing child needs proteins. Proteins can be obtained from pulses, grains, milk and milk products. Eggs, fish, meat also make diet rich in proteins. However, scientific studies have shown that non-vegetarian diet taken regularly predisposes to high cholesterol level, high blood pressure and malignancy of intestines. It is believed that people on vegetarian diet remain healthier and live longer. Today, there is an increasing preference for a vegetarian diet.

Vitamins

They are an essential part of a balanced diet. Our body and brain need a number of vitamins. Green vegetables, fruits, fish, meat and egg are quite rich in vitamins. Craze for taking fast foods is catching in urban India. Medical experts call it junk food. It is rich in calories, but poor in balanced nutrition. By taking, cakes, noodles, chocolates or cold drinks one may get sufficient calories, but one loses appetite and remains deficient in vitamins and other essential nutritions. It has been proved in many places that such diet can lead to malnourishment. In the USA, scientists have found that children coming from Asian homes eating traditional diets, are healthier than American children. Non-nutritious diet is going to decrease your capacity to face a stressful situation. So, a balanced and nutritious diet is the best defense for day-to-day physical and mental stresses.

CONCLUSION

It is important to realize that depression is a state of human mind and our mind is always subjected to so many pulls and pressures and when such pressures become too much for a given person, one tends to break down. But the most promising part is that most of the cases of depression show complete recovery without any remnant scars, so during a phase of depression, when everything looks dark and gloomy, sustaining a hope and a bright hope in the Almighty is the finest ladder to come out of the mess.

10

Skin Care: Part of Total Fitness

Adarsh Chopra* and Dimple Chopra**

Skin is the largest organ of the body. Besides giving shape and expression to the body it has many other functions to perform: (1) It protects our body from the adverse effects of sun and environment, (2) Act as a mechanical barrier and does not allow any outside organisms to stay or penetrate into the skin as it being constantly shed-off, (3) In the presence of sun it synthesizes vitamin D3, (4) It regulates the body temp. and proportions of salt in the body by sweat. Besides all these functions in general glowing shiny skin is a sign of beauty and it plays an important role in social communication. So it becomes our foremost duty to take care of it and keep it glowing shiny supple and wrinkle free without any pigmentation or scars.

Skin has two basic components—Epidermis (Outer) and Dermis (Inner) and two appendages—hairs, nails and two glands—sebaceous and sweat glands (eccrine and apocrine). Any damage to dermis and below will lead to scar formation while any injury over the epidermis does not leave any scar.

* (Ex) Professor of Skin and V.D., Government Medical College, Patiala.

** Dermatologist.

The concept of skin care has undergone significant changes over the last few years in India because of increased awareness and availability of various cosmetics and advertisement media.

Daily skin care depends upon the local climatic conditions, nature of person's duty, activity and the skin type. Usually the skin types are:

1. Dry Skin

Dry skin is that which looks dry and improves by the applications of emolients. It gives matty and dull appearance along with dry and rough feel to touch. Sometimes it results in visible scaling, association with dandruff and/or may be associated with irritation, redness and itching and rarely cracks over more mobile areas like angles of the mouth and heels. Fingers of the working hands get dry and fissured, so this type of skin needs more attention and care.

2. Oily Skin

It is a greasy and shiny to look at. It is because of the excessive secretion of sebum and/or excessive use of greasy cosmetics. Sometimes it gives a pulpy coating. Enlarged pores and acne usually accompany the oily skin.

3. Normal Skin

This is an ideal skin type with sufficient sebum and moisture necessary to keep it soft and supple; so that it gives neither oily nor dry look.

There are a few simple basics required to look after the skin.

1. Diet
2. Exercise
3. Local skin care—
   (a) Skin of face, body and body folds
   (b) Hands and feet
   (c) Hair care
   (d) Nail care

Diet

There are a few myths about skin and food. Some believe that fish along with milk and or white food causes vitiligo or spicy and fried food give rise to pimples but this is Not True, skin requires a well balanced diet consisting of milk, curd, cheese, green vegetables, eggs, etc.

Exercise

Regular walking, jogging, cycling, is an important factor to keep the skin shiny and healthy. On the back of all these a healthy, positive thinking mind is an important factor as it goes with the old saying, "Face is the index of mind" so if we think good and positive our skin will show the same.

Skin care has three basic principles:

- ❑ Cleansing
- ❑ Toning
- ❑ Moisturising

Usually soaps are used for skin cleansing bathing, washing of hands and hair. Types of soaps used varies according to the economical status and personal liking of the colour and fragrances but it should be according to skin type. There are superfatted soaps with more of oil and fat which are good for dry skin. Transparent soaps having glycerine and little of sucrose are good for all skins. Acne soaps are used if the persons have pimples. Normal skin persons can use any soap provided it does not cause allergy. Bath should be taken twice daily. Liquid soaps or cleansing milks can also be used as an alternate or along with soaps.

Facial skin being more delicate, many prefer to use the alternatives over the face as facial packs, foams and gels or cleansing milk, tiny particles of rough, granulated material like orange peal with mild detergents. Old traditional Basin + Haldi + Cream + Water is very useful for dry and normal skin.

Dry Skin

Soaps for dry skin should be superfatted soaps with more of oil. Glycerin-based soaps, cleansing milks, liquid paraffin, cold creams are to be used to make it supple while moisturizing agents should be used to maintain the water content of the epidermis and keep body moist.

Oily Skin

Oily skin persons should use non-glycerin soap. Abrasive cleansers are to be used on the face hands and arms and should be used twice or thrice daily. Dusting and talc powder will be of help.

Toning

Toning is an essential part after cleansing especially for the facial skin. Toners are available in various concentration of alcohol to suit the skin types. Oily skin needs more of alcohol content while dry skin needs no toning or toning with more of water content.

Moisturising

In our country it is essential to use moisturizers because heat, pollution, sunrays, etc. combine to make the skin dry. Using moisturizers at night and sun screen during the day will protect the skin to a great extent. The softness, suppleness, resilience and pliability of skin depends upon the water content of the skin. Various types of moisturising agents are available like cold creams, night creams, lotions, and other medicated moisturising agents. For normal skin oil in water moisturizers are preferred during night and lotions in the day time, while in dry skin more of water in oil should be used along with the moisturizers and emolients. In oily skin these should be avoided.

Traditional oil massage before bath, works as an emollient. Bathing with curd, curd milk is very useful especially for the head bath as it use to work as a toner and emollient. These are helpful for dry and normal skin. Another specialized use of moisturizers as a protectant against daily sun light by incorporating the sunscreens and anti-aging effect by addition of glycolic acid.

Dusting

In tropical country like India, talcum powder is used as

dusting agent after bath in intertriginous areas like axillae, groins and finger webs as it absorbs sweat and prevent infection and friction. Deodorants are also used but sometimes they cause allergy and skin becomes thickened and hyperpigmented after their prolonged use.

Hair

Long hair is a tradition in India. The scalp and the hair are soiled by dust and this dust is held on by a film of greasy sebum and forms adhesions of greasy hair resulting in itching and falling of hair. Normal hair care aims at keeping the scalp and hair free from dust and excess grease by washing/shampooing twice weekly and avoiding heat drying, combing wet hair excessively, colouring and perming as they lead to hair loss especially from hair shaft.

Hands and Feet

Hands and feet are daily exposed to irritants which may be chemical or physical agents during usual working at home and/or at job. Cumulative insults results in the removing of protective lipid layer resulting in dry, red, lusterless dry hands. We can avoid it by reducing the frequency of washing hands, use of mild and better detergents and use of lotions. Hand lotions containing water, oil or creams of same nature or petrolatum jelly, will be of help especially if used after soaking the hands for 5-20 min. in luke warm water. Special care should be taken of finger webs as they remain wet and moist giving rise to infections. So they should be dried after every washing and moisturizing agents are to be massaged. In summer dusting powder should be used to keep the area dry.

Feet

Usually closed shoes are used by men and open chappals by women at work while at home only open chappals are used. Throughout the day closed shoes causes discomfort and repeated insults to feet causing dermatitis, thickening and ultimately fissuring. To keep the feet good looking and comfortable one must massage the feet with oil before bathing in the morning and while putting on socks one should spray some powder in finger webs. While at night soak the feet in luke warm water, rub with steel wool or pumice stone followed by the application of emollients like jelly or moisturizers and do some massage which will keep the feet fissure free.

Nails

Require additional attention as they are mainly meant for protection of fingertips but they are also important for cosmetic manipulation. Repeated injuries and insults to nails lead to chipped, thin, brittle, lusterless and bad shaped nails. We can keep them shining by the application of moisturizers, hand lotions containing water in oil or creams of same nature or petroleum jelly, after soaking the hands of feet for 5-10 minutes in luke warm water. Soft brush should be used to remove the foreign material under the nails. Nails should be cut with the sharp scissors and never with teeth. Cuticle should not be damaged while brushing or cutting there wise it will lead to infection.

Keeping these points in view we can protect our skin from premature aging wrinkling and pigmentation, etc. and keep it shiny, supple and good looking.

11

Healthy Teeth and Gums: Insurance to Fitness of Body System

VIRESH CHOPRA* AMD HIMANSHU AERAN**

The most common dental diseases are periodontal disease, gum disease and dental caries or commonly known as tooth decay. Now-a-days due to the enhanced use of tobacco, pan masala, gutka, the incidence of oral cancer is also increasing day by day. We will try to explain what you should know about all these three conditions.

GUM DISEASE

What is Periodontal Disease?

A disease that affects the gums and other supporting structures of the teeth is known as Periodontal disease. It is commonly known as gum disease. The early stage of this disease is referred to as Gingivitis and is characterised by inflammed gums which bleed easily. In the more advanced stage the disease affects the bone and other supporting structures and is known as periodontitis.

---

* BDS, Dental Surgeon.

** MDS, Professor & Vice-Principal, Subharati Dental College, Meerut.

What Causes Gum Disease?

The early stage of gum disease, gingivitis, starts with plaque. Plaque is a soft, sticky colourless film of bacteria that constantly forms on teeth. If you do not clean your teeth properly, the plaque builds up and the bacteria produce toxins and enzymes that can irritate the gums. Gums can become red, swollen, sensitive and can bleed on provocation.

How do you Know if you have it?

Some early warning signs of impending gum disease are:

Gingivitis	Red, swollen or tender gums, gums that bleed while brushing.
Periodontitis	Gums separated from your teeth. Pus between teeth and gums. Change in the way teeth fit together. Loose or shifting teeth. Bad breath or bad taste.

Should you notice any of the above sign and symptoms, visit your dentist immediately.

What Happens if Gingivitis is not Treated?

In time, the build-up of plaque can move below the gum-line. This causes an inflammation, which forms pockets, that is a space between the teeth and gums. It also destroys the underlying bone. This advanced stage is known as periodontitis. As more bone gets destroyed, the tooth can loosen and eventually fall out or may need to be removed.

Who can get Gum Disease?

Although periodontal disease can occur at any age, they usually affect adults. As many as 90% of people above 40 years suffer from some form of gum-disease, making it the leading cause of tooth loss in adults.

How can you Prevent Gingivitis?

- ❑ The only effective way is to prevent build-up of plaque. Brushing and flossing twice a day and after meals can control plaque build-up.

- ❑ Eat a balanced diet, especially one rich in dietary fiber. Fresh fruit and vegetables, milk and fish are recommended.
- ❑ Visit your dentist at least twice a year. He is trained to recognize early symptoms of gum disease and offer curative procedures.

So Gum Disease is Curable?

Yes, Early gingivitis is usually completely reversible. Your dentist will treat the disease through professional cleaning and scaling to remove plaque. You must follow that up with certain preventive measures that prevent the resettling of plaque at the gum-line.

Advanced gum disease, now referred to as periodontitis, may require surgery to help save teeth. Only very advanced stages are incurable.

How do you Prevent the Onset of Gum Disease in the First Place?

Certain preventive measures are known to prevent the re-settling of plaque at the gum-line and therefore, reduce the risk of gum disease. You must practice these good dental habits.

Brushing

Brush your teeth twice a day. Hold a soft brush at the gum line at a 45° angle. Brush in a circular notion to massage the gums and an up-down motion to dislodge plaque. Do this gently on the outer as well as inner surfaces of teeth.

Replace your brush every 2 or 3 months.

Floss

Floss daily to remove plaque from between teeth. Take about 18" of floss and wrap most of it around your middle finger and the rest around the middle finger of the other hand, leaving a 2" length between them. Using your thumb and forefinger, gently scrape the side of each tooth away from the gum.

Rinse

Rinse your mouth with water thoroughly after each meal. Rinse for a minute everyday with mouthwash.

DENTAL CARIES

What is Tooth Decay?

Tooth Decay describes the condition wherein the tooth, under a variety of harsh conditions, break down leading to the formation of a cavity. It starts with a hole/opening in the enamel. If this is not treated, it progressively reaches the deeper sections of the tooth, where the pulp and the nerves are causing the tooth to become sensitive to a variety of stimuli, a variety of gum problems such as inflammation and swelling, pain and ultimately tooth loss.

Is it Very Common?

Tooth decay is a common dental ailment that may occur at any time or age. However, since the onset of tooth decay is strongly related to the unregulated consumption of sweet foods and beverages, it tends to affect the young and adolescents more than any other age. One form is diagnosed in nursing infants and is referred to a nursing caries.

What is Baby Bottle Tooth Decay?

A serious form of tooth decay affects nursing infants and is called "Nursing caries" or "Baby bottle tooth decay." In infants who are nursed continuously with a bottle/formula milk/pacifiers; the milk is retained in the mouth as the child falls asleep with the bottle. This milk is an excellent nutritive media for a variety of germs present in the mouth. The milk is broken down by the germs to form harsh acids which lead to the formation of a cavity on the tooth.

What are the Causes of Tooth Decay?

1. Poor Oral Hygiene

Irregular and improper brushing, not flossing between teeth, not rinsing with water or mouthwash after meals speed up the process of tooth decay.

2. Unregulated Diet of Sweet Food

Periodic snacking on aerated drinks, jam, marmalade, even potato chips can lead to the formation of acidic by products which damage the surface of the tooth enamel. This is the reason why most young children adolescents suffer from tooth decay.

3. Bad or Worn out Dental Fillings

Tooth decay might develop again from exposed tooth surfaces.

What can you do if you have Tooth Decay?

If you have developed black or brown spots of decay on your teeth either in the fissures or on the smooth surfaces and it is associated with discomfort and/or sensitivity to hot and cold and/or frank pain, it is likely that you have tooth decay. Your dentist will evaluate you comprehensively and based on his clinical and radiographic findings he will do one of the followings:

1. Make on opening in the crown and remove decay, shape the cavity and fill it with a tooth coloured filling or an amalgam filling. This could also be done under local anaesthesia.
2. If the decay is very deep and the pulp (nerve, root canal) is involved in the decay process he will, under local anaesthesia go deeper into the pulp chamber, remove the pulp and the nerve, render it free of infection, do a root filling and later put an amalgam or a tooth coloured filling. Subsequently he will put a veneer or a crown on the tooth as the case may be.

Prevention is the Best Cure for Tooth Decay

Certain preventive measures are known to reduce the risk of tooth decay. You must practice these good dental habits.

Brushing

Brush your teeth twice a day. Hold a soft brush at the

gum line at a 45° angle. Brush in a circular motion to massage the gums and an up-down motion to dislodge plaque. Do this gently on the outer as well as inner surfaces of teeth.

Choose the Right Tooth Brush

Dentists recommend using a toothbrush with soft bristles and a small head. Replace your toothbrush every 3 months or as soon as it loses it's original shape. Once a brush loses its shape, you require more pressure for the same cleaning action. This extra pressure is damaging to gums as well as the protective enamel layer.

Floss

Floss daily to remove plaque from between teeth. Take about 18" of floss and wrap most of it around your middle finger and the rest around the middle finger of the other hand, leaving a 2" length between them. Using your thumb and forefinger, gently scrape the side of each tooth away from the gum.

Rinse

Rinse your mouth with water thoroughly after each meal. May Rinse for a minute everyday mouthwash.

Diet

Reducing the frequency of intake of sweets during the day, decreases the number of 'acid attack' by the digestive breakdown to these foods in the mouth. This prevents further damage to the tooth.

Expectant mothers must be particularly careful with their diet and must make sure that it contains all the necessary nutrients and vitamins (described below) since the foundation of a child's teething is laid early in the second trimester (3 to 6 months).

A balanced diet that includes all food groups such as fresh fruits, vegetables, bread, cereals as well as other grain products. Dairy products such as milk, cheese, yogurt, meat, poultry, fish provides the essential nutrients required for dental growth. (See Appendix IV: 'Oral Health' for further details, as adopted by World Health assembly).

ORAL CANCER

What is Oral Cancer?

Oral Cancer is a disease that starts as an uncontrolled growth of cells in the mouth. It leads to disfigurement of the face, debility of body and eventually death.

Is it Very Common?

Oral Cancer is the most common of cancers in India with as many as 64,460 cases reported each year. That makes it as common as cancer of the lungs, breast or cervix. As much as 7% of all cancer deaths in males and 4% in females have been reported to be due to oral cancer. The figure continues to rise rapidly because of bad oral habits such as chewing of gutka, tobacco and smoking among people of all age groups.

What are the Early Warning Signs?

A white or red patch in the mouth or on the tongue, a painless ulcer which doesn't heal for over two weeks, difficulty in eating, drinking and speaking are some of the early signs of oral cancer. If these symptoms appear, you must see your dentist immediately.

Can you Examine yourself?

Yes, you can. In fact, it is strongly recommended because early detection can greatly increase the chances of a complete cure—

- ❑ Stand in front of a mirror in good light.
- ❑ Open your mouth wide. Look for small lumps or swelling, ulcers, a red or white patch.
- ❑ If you have dentures, take them out and inspect your mouth.
- ❑ Inspect the lips with your mouth both open and closed.
- ❑ Stick your tongue out and inspect the margins, as well as below the tongue.
- ❑ If you see something abnormal visit your dentist immediately.

What are the Early Clinical Indicators?

A good dentist is trained to recognize the clinical symptoms of an early oral cancer:

Leukoplakia

It is a raised white patch, which may be associated with the constant chewing of tobacco and gutka. 2.8% of oral Leukoplakia results in cancerous growths.

Oral Submucous Fibrosis

It is the inability or difficulty to open the mouth and/ or a burning sensation which affects 9 per 10,000 Indians.

Lichen Planus

It is skin affliction occurring in the mouth. It can be caused due to stress and diabetes.

Anaemia

It is a deficiency of iron very common in India, which can lead to the development of oral cancer.

Can Oral Cancer be Cured? How?

If detected early, oral cancer is curable. The smaller the ulcer of affliction, the better the chances of cure.

Treatment involves the surgical removal of the afflicted parts followed by radiation. Chemotherapy is rarely advocated. Cancer of the lip shows 85% cure-rate. Other oral cancers if detected early and treated promptly, may prolong the life of the patients, by as much as 20 year.

How to Avoid Oral Cancer?

Since oral cancer is very common in India, extra precaution is suggested—

- Avoid bad oral habits like chewing tobacco, gutka and smoking. These bad habits increase your chances of getting oral cancer dramatically.
- Eat a diet rich in fiber, fresh fruits and vegetables, fish and dairy products such as butter milk.
- Visit your dentist twice a year.
- Brush twice a day and maintain good oral hygiene.

12

How to Guide Patients Suffering from Life Threatening Probelms

RANJIV MITTAL*

Patients suffering from long standing life-threatening problems suffer on two counts. One is due to the disease, its symptoms, side effects of drugs, uncertainty of their life, and other problems associated with hospital treatment like long queues, shortage of men and material, inadequate financial resources, paper work etc.

The other one is that he is a silent and suffering spectator who has no idea what is being done to his body and in what way he can participate in his healing process. How can he utilize his mental and physical energy in a way that will make him a part the team interested in bringing him back to health. Doctors are only interested that he should submit to their interventions meekly and allow them to deal with his body like an experimental animal. There are lots of studies which indicate that participation on the part of the patient can make a major difference in the outcome of treatment in the form of cure or prolongation of life. The

* Çonsultant, Holistic Health, Chandigarh.

work of Dr. Bernie Siegal in this area is an example. He is giving conventional treatment to his cancer patients like surgery, chemotherapy, radiotherapy. Along with these conventional treatments he is asking them to do visualization. Dr. Bernie's patients are the longest surviving in the world. The study of Dr. Spiegel on breast cancer patients, Norman Coussins self-cure, Kathryn Shafer's self-cure of asthma by creative visualization, Robert Dilts work with her mother resulting in the cure of her metastasized breast cancer without any conventional treatment are all powerful examples which indicate that involvement of patient in the healing process is not only useful but essential and mandatory to complete the healing process. Dr. Dean Ornish's work in the reversal of the heart disease can be taken as a module for guiding the patients in how can they participate in their own treatment.

The patients are to be guided in the following areas:

1. Understanding one's own self.
2. Understanding and interacting with others.
3. Connecting with a higher self.
4. Changing one's beliefs, identity, capabilities, environment and behaviour.
5. Specific techniques for the treatment of different diseases.
6. Creating specific support groups where patients can visit regularly.
7. Creating tangible targets for the patients to achieve.

Understanding Self

(A) Yoga

Although many people feel that Yoga is only a collection of various stretching exercises and postures to limber up the body, it is more than that. Yoga includes breathing techniques, meditation, visualization, progressive relaxation practices, self-analysis, altruism. All of these methods have one common purpose, i.e. to our isolation. Yoga is a set of powerful set of tools for achieving union—

and healing—with parts of ourselves. Awareness is the first step in healing. Our attention is drawn outwards from morning till night. We seldom take time to notice what is on inside our own body or mind until something goes wrong and we are in pain. Increasing our awareness extends our control over what is happening within. As we can notice the effects of stress: tension, conflicts, negative beliefs much earlier and make changes before they become full blown illness such as heart disease and cancer, etc. All of these exercises have one common purpose and that is to help quiet one's mind and body, thus enabling us to experience a sense of relaxation, peace and joy.

Relaxation and lethargy are not the same. Our body and mind function most efficiently and effectively when we are relaxed. It is not always possible to avoid external stress but it is possible to change our reaction to it.

Stretching

The first step towards experiencing inner peace and healing is to quiet down and relax the body which in turn quietens the mind. The various techniques are:

(a) Head rotations.
(b) Shoulder shrugs.
(c) Twists.
(d) Back stretch (Cobra pose).
(e) Leg lift (half and full locust).
(f) Forward stretch with both legs.
(g) Forward stretch with single leg alternately.
(h) Shoulder stand.
(i) Chest extension.
(j) Half spinal twist.
(k) Forward stretch in lotus.
(l) Sun salutation (Surya namskar).
(m) Resting position (shav posture).

Progressive Muscular Relaxation

Different persons use different variations of this method but basic steps remain same. These steps are:

(1) Tense different groups of muscles one by one and experience that feeling of stretch in the mind.
(2) Relax different groups of muscles one by one and experience that feeling of relaxation of each muscle group in the mind.
(3) Sometimes the feeling of relaxation feels profoundly healing on many levels. Thoughts, feelings that were previously walled-off may come to the surface, where they can be reintegrated into one's awareness. Just notice whatever thoughts or feelings come up, but let then pass without trying to judge, suppress, or control them.
(4) Bring your awareness to your breathing. Without trying to change the pattern of your breathing, just feel the gentle flow of air as it comes in and out of your nose.
(5) After a moment or when you desire gradually allow your inhalations to become little deeper with each breath. Imagine that you are breathing in light and healing energy as well as oxygen that is revitalizing and recharging your body and mind.
(6) After spending some time in this state, slowly move toes, fingers, hands and feet and slowly opening the eyes come into the sitting position.
(7) After you have practiced the deep relaxation several times, you may be able to get into this state without having to sequentially tense and relax each group of muscle.

BREATHING TECHNIQUES (PRANAYAMA)

Your breath is a bridge between your body and mind. Changes in your body affect your breathing, for example during exercise.

Changes in your mind affect your breathing. When you are anxious, your breathing is rapid and shallow. When you are relaxed you breathe slower and deeper. Reverse is also true. Changes in your breathing affect your mind and body profoundly. Besides this your breathing is a bridge between the sympathetic and parasympathetic nervous system. These breathing techniques when practiced regularly produce a profound calming effect on your mind and body and decrease sympathetic nervous simulation.

These breathing techniques also called pranayama can expand and balance the availability and flow of vital energy (Prana). By combining this with other techniques you can learn to direct this energy to assist in the process of health and healing. In other words, your emotional state affects your breathing, which in turn affects your energy, body and that affects the physical body.

One of the ways we respond to stress is by holding our breath. Over time when the stress is chronic, this disturbance in the flow of vital energy can lead to life threatening disturbances.

(1) Abdominal breathing.
(2) Yogic deep breathing.
(3) Bellows breathing.
(4) Alternate nostril breathing.

VISUALISATION

One of the characteristics of the sub-conscious mind is that it does not differentiate between strong imagination and reality. Visualization is a very and most effective method to focus your s/c mind on any thing you wish to achieve. Consequently if you can learn to focus your s/c mind on healing and recovery you can achieve that because s/c mind is nine times stronger and is in charge of involuntary processes going on in our body like working of immune system, maintaining blood pressure, athrogenesis and balancing the tone of sympathetic and parasympathetic system. Our mind talks to your body by using mental images. This communication is going on all the time—sometimes in healing ways, sometimes in harmful ways—although most of the time you are not aware of it. This communication happens best when all the five senses are used in imagination. Under the heading visualization two processes are most common. The first is directed visualization and the other is receptive visualization.

(i) Directed Visualization

As you have completed progressive muscular relaxation then imagine that you are dealing the disease you are suffering from using all your five senses. You can create different imagery for different disease. For example, you can create an erection of the penis by visualization which is just an increase of blood flow in the penile artery.

By same analogy you can increase the blood flow in the coronary artery by your thoughts. Similar visualizations can be constructed for other diseases like Kauravas being killed by Pandavas in case of cancer and so on. One can learn this technique of directed visualization in a matter of one to two weeks.

(ii) Receptive Visualization

Using receptive visualization, you can bring to your conscious mind useful information that had been unconscious or ignored. Instead of choosing a mental image that you want to occur, you receive images from your mind that arise in response to your questions. Receptive visualization is based on the idea that you know more about yourself than you may be aware of. Dr. Dean Ornish who has worked with many heart patients is amazed at how frequently a similar image of a wall or fortress around the heart appears from a person's s/c.

Using imagery you can begin a dialogue with these inner parts of ourselves. If the world is a dangerous place and if the expressions of feelings is dangerous, then it may seem easier not to feel at all. You will need to keep your heart closed and isolated. If you put up walls to protect the scared child that you may have within yourselves—this child that feels unworthy, not quite good enough or attractive enough to be loved, or incapable of handling the world around, or feels no longer useful in this world—it is really hard to begin this process of opening up. Connecting with inner deep rooted feelings is the beginning of the healing process in life threatening diseases. One of the ways of doing receptive visualization is called INNER TEACHER VISUALIZATION. Another way of doing this in case of heart patients is called THE INNER HEART VISUALIZATIONS.

These yoga techniques—stretching, progressive muscular relaxation, breathing and visualization—are powerful tools for stress management and healing.

UNDERSTANDING AND INTERACTING WITH OTHERS

It is not only what we are doing, it is how we approach what we are doing that determines if we end up feeling more connected to others or more alone. Some actions are more intensely charged than others and so have more energy to push us in either direction. To the lovers sexual relationship is the most uniting and transcendent experience while survivors of rape experience profound feelings of isolation and difficulty in trusting. Similarly, death can be viewed as going into a dark room, all alone, forever—the ultimate isolating experience. Or it can be a transcendent experience, a return to the source. How we approach other people each day can determine whether we experience isolation, chronic stress, suffering and illness or intimacy, relaxation, joy and health. Touching, hugging and massage are ways of increasing intimacy under appropriate conditions. Three powerful techniques are:

- ❑ Communication skills.
- ❑ Altruism, compassion and forgiveness.
- ❑ Group support and sharing secrets.

Communication Skills

When we feel heard we feel more connected.

Ventilation

Ventilation is just getting your feelings out; you really do not care whether the person hears you or not.

Communication

Communication is expressing how you feel to someone so that he or she can hear and understand you better. It is a learnable skill. Basic principle of good communication is that our feelings help to connect us, whereas thoughts—especially judgments—tend to isolate us. Our emotions are more likely to be heard than our thoughts. Communicating ideas brings our minds together, whereas communicating emotions unites our hearts—not quite the same experience.

(a) Thoughts are much more likely to be heard as criticisms than are feelings.
(b) As soon as feel criticized by someone, it is hard to hear anything else he or she has to say.
(c) Feelings are true statements.
(d) Listening is not the same as obeying.
(e) Expressing feelings seems to make us a little vulnerable, although it really makes us safer.
(f) Feelings are more powerful than thoughts at influencing us.
(g) Expressing feelings helps to keep the discussion in the present moment.
(h) Step Learning to express feelings.

Step I

Identify what you are feeling. It is not that easy as it sounds. Many people have a hard time telling the difference between a thought and a feeling. Feelings are expressed as I am—angry, afraid, worried, thrilled, confused, happy, depressed, envious, resentful or I love you or I want—.

Some common thoughts/judgments are:

I am right.
You are wrong.
You are not listening.
You did it again.
You are always late.
You forgot.
You should wear different clothes.

Words like "you should", "you ought to", "you never" and "you always" are thoughts and heard as judgments or criticisms.

Step 2

Express what you are feeling.

Say what you feel, express it as a feeling whether positive or negative but not as thought or judgment. This helps to break the vicious cycle of attack, counter-attack and withdrawal.

Step 3

Listen actively with empathy and compassion. Knowing how to listen is as important a communication skill as knowing how to express feelings. Try to hear the feelings in what the other person is saying, even if he or she is not expressing it clearly or expressing it as a judgment. Remember that the other person wants to feel heard, just as you do. You are not always going to get the other person to agree with you, but at least you will understand each other better. Opening, listening and giving one's attention help to bring us together. Compassion and empathy are healing.

Empathy and sympathy are not same. Empathy means listening with compassion—trying to understand what the other person is feeling. Sympathy means feeling sorry for someone, a usually well-intentioned gesture that often creates more distance between people. The unspoken message can be "You are the one with the problem, not me."

A variant of sympathy is giving unsolicited advice. When we hear someone describing a problem, our tendency is to try to fix it by jumping in with our own advice, comments, criticisms or experiences. Often the other person just wants to feel listened to and understood, which leads to greater intimacy even when the problem is not easily solvable. The unspoken message behind unsolicited advice can be "I know the answer; how come you do not?" Creating more distance and less intimacy. Listening is very often more supportive a response than giving someone advice.

Step 4

Acknowledge what the other person is saying. Understanding the other person does not mean that you agree with him. Saying "I want" is a clear and direct feeling—no one can argue with it if it is true or not. And it makes you a little more vulnerable and open, since the other person knows he or she can disappoint you by not giving you what you want. Therefore saying, "I want" is something most of us are taught to avoid. In fact, "I want" is a clear and most direct way to avoid the other person feeling manipulated. And when we feel manipulated or controlled, we do not feel free. When we try to control or manipulate someone, he or she usually resents it. More than being healthy we want to feel free, and we cannot feel free when we are being controlled. Doctors refer to a patient's compliance as if the patient is surrendering his will and freedom to the doctor. GOD made the mistake of manipulating Adam and Eve when He told them not to eat Apple. And human beings said, "Why not" or "Why me." We are carrying on the same trait since then.

ALTRUISM, COMPASSION AND FORGIVENESS

Altruism, compassion and forgiveness—opening your heart—can be powerful means of healing the isolation that leads to stress, suffering and illness. In other words, these are in our own interest, for they help to free us from our limitations and empower us. A study of 2754 people followed up to twelve years revealed that men who did no volunteer work were two and a half times more likely to die during the study period compared to men who volunteered at least once a week. These results were independent of age, sex or health status when they first entered the study. Acting selflessly is the most selfish way to behave since it maintains our inner sense of peace and joy. Compassion and forgiveness are empowering and healing both for the giver and the recipient. By remaining compassionate, we can stop binding ourselves and limiting our freedom. We might live longer but we will live better.

GROUP SUPPORT/SHARING SECRETS

There is a fundamental paradox: when we have the courage to be self-disclosing, to show who we really are—then other people in the group feel safer to show who they really are, too. This allows us to experience new levels of intimacy rather than rejection and isolation. But if you never have any place that you feel safe enough to show who you really are, anyone with whom you can really be yourself, then it is ultimately stressful and isolating.

Summary

Use the communication skills to express feelings from your heart without being judgmental.

Create a support group or join an existing one that feels safe enough for you to let down your walls, take-off your masks, and show your true self.

Doing well may be good for you, under the right circumstances. Make a point of helping others in ways that you choose and that feel comfortable for you.

We can use our pain—emotional or physical—as a catalyst to begin healing, not just curing. Curing means only getting back to the way we were before we became diseased. Healing is when we use our pain or illness as a catalyst to begin transforming our lives—healing our inner pain and our relationships, our hearts and our souls.

CONNECTING WITH A HIGHER SELF

Our senses of perception are directed outwards. In the childhood we are trained to perceive outside objects. How this process happens inside us remains at the sub-conscious (s/c) level. Creating awareness of sensations happening inside us takes a little longer and also how to control them. To learn to control passing of urine and stools takes a little longer time. Similarly, controlling the flow of inputs from outside is easier as it is easier to block the senses from outside that is by closing our eyes, ears, nose, etc. The processing of this information takes place outside our conscious awareness therefore, it is little difficult to create awareness about this. In a way our senses of perception are habituated to experience outside world. To create awareness about inside pictures, dialogue, sensations, smells and tastes is what is called the beginning of meditation. Once this awareness is created then the next phase starts and that is to minimize this deluge of different sensations. Then the next phase starts and that is to give direction so that awareness is focused in the desired and smaller area. The last phase is then to create a sensationless state, which leads to a complete transformation of the individual irreversibly which has been differently described as samadhi, zen, no mind or union with the self, etc.

HOW TO MEDITATE

Meditation is of different types. A simple and powerful method is:

- ❑ Sit comfortably in an alert but relaxed posture and practice to remain motionless for atleast half an hour.
- ❑ Focus on your breathing.
- ❑ Focusing on a sound. (Religious or secular)
- ❑ Mindfulness.
- ❑ Self-analysis.
- ❑ Prayer or devotion.

The whole purpose of meditation is to quiten the mind by different techniques and then experience that inner silence. Once this inner silence is experienced the integration of conscious and s/c mind takes place, the conflicts are removed and a complete transformation of personality takes place. Different religions differ in this method of quitening the mind, the end result being the same in each case. Most of the times we become entangled in the rituals that were created for giving the followers clear guidelines to start this process of achieving inner harmony and quietness. Each saint or seer reached this transformation in his own way and taught the same process to his followers. Grasping the essence of the technique and then applying it as per one's own inclinations is the fundamental of this path. Insisting that one's own path is the only right path and all other paths are not only childish but also dangerous. This stubbornness has caused so much bitterness and enimosity amongst various religious groups.

The posture recommended in general is that one should sit with the maximum base firmly based on the ground and keeping the vertebral column erect and perpendicular to the ground. Legs should be kept in a posture, which causes minimum of strain. Folding the legs has a physiological effect in the sense that in that pose the least amount of blood will be flowing to the lower half of the body and naturally larger amount of blood is available for the brain. The body is relaxed in that posture. Relaxation of the muscles revitalizes the cells and this is achieved by progressive muscular relaxation or thought massage. It means that the meditator with closed eyes sends his thoughts consciously down his body, carefully massaging and relaxing every muscle. In this position of relaxation, you will be putting-off the physical body as it were on a cross-represented by vertebral column and the shoulder blades. It is noteworthy that the strength of one's meditation does not depend on the kind of seat or the quality of mattress, etc. Once we have learnt the art of meditation one can meditate any where and under all circumstances. It was discovered by ancient seers that the unit of life is an experience. On the analysis of a single experience it was realized that a combination of three is required, the experiencer, the experienced and the experiencing. Ancient seers took the world of subject as their area of study that is the experiencer. In a superficial observation it was noticed that each one of us has four distinct entities, each demanding its own satisfaction. These are physical, mental, intellectual and spiritual. This four headed hydra thus seeks its own satisfaction by drinking from a single cup when it has four parched throats, each demanding for its satisfaction a different beverage altogether. Satisfaction of one of them leads to the dissatisfaction of the others as many times the demands seem conflicting. Deeper the layer which is satisfied, more effective it is in achieving longer happiness. Mental happiness is more durable than physical one, intellectual is better than mental and spiritual is everlasting.

The study of the experiencer led to different states of awareness that is waking state, the dream state, and the deep sleep state. Man undergoes different impressions during these three states of conscious. These impressions appear real when we are in that state of conscious but appear unreal when our state of conscious changes. Experiences of the deep sleep state appear unreal in dream state and that of dream state in wakeful state and *vice-versa*. The world, which is perceived by five senses of perception, is a state of consciousness, called wakeful state. When we identify with our subtle body and look into inner experiences, this is called dream state. Withdrawal from both wakeful and dream state into deep sleep is a different state. When we transgress these three states, we come to discover the spiritual entity, the illuminating factor, the divine spark, and the life center the TURIYA state. Meditation is a process by which we reach this state of self-discovery.

Mind

Just as water flowing continuously in one direction in a river, so too thought flow is the mind. Just as the continuous flow of gallons of water gives us the magnitude of the river, thoughts flowing continuously from an individual towards the world of objects, is the mind. The nature and behaviour of thought in an individual bosom at a given moment must condition and define the type of mind the individual possesses at that time. The transformation of mind requires change in the quality, the quantity and the direction of thought-flow. The quality of thoughts in our mind will depend upon the type of objects that initiate or sustain the nature of thoughts within the company of good books, noble men and surrendering himself to the Lord that is *bhakti* are the means by which the quality of thoughts can be improved.

Quantity of thoughts are caused by: (1) shackling memories of the past, (2) benumbing fears of the past, (3) freezing anxieties with the present changes taking place around. Selfless dedicated activity undertaken as an offering in a spirit of surrender to the Lord is the only available method to control this flood of thoughts. The direction of thoughts is changed by the pursuit of knowledge of infinite Self that expresses itself through the vehicles of body, mind and intellect. In short, the paths of devotion (*bhakti*), action (*karma*) and knowledge (*jnana*) are to be practiced in synthesis. Hence, the importance of Japa yoga, where in all the three come into play.

JAPA YOGA

Japa is a training of the mind in fixing itself to a single line of thinking. The mind of the seeker is made single pointed by practicing the recital of a sound/mantra sitting at the feet of the Lord. Mind is a delusory thing which seems to have potency and power where thoughts are flowing. When thoughts parade in our intellect and march out, one after another, in a continuous and unbroken stream, we have the delusory idea or feeling that there is a substantial phantom of mighty power and irresistible threat called the mind. Meditation is a process by which the meditator entertains his entire mind in the contemplation of a series of similar thought currents to the exclusion of all dissimilar thought intrusions, so that he may ultimately minimize his thoughts to the bare possible minimum of a single idea.

The chanting of mantra/sound is first done loudly. After the loud chanting, start the mental chanting. When the lips are closed, we are not to stop chanting but continue within. Let the mind chant on. But after a week or so you will find that mind can chant freely but it can wander into worldly fields of activity. At such moments let your intellect order the mind to chant on a maximum pitch. Let this chanting continue till mental fatigue is felt. Then suddenly halt the chanting and experience a moment of divine silence. This state of silence is a state of transcendence of the mind. The longer the interval that one can create between the moment one has stopped chanting and the moment the first thought enters the more shall one feel full empty existence. In the ground thus prepared seeds of positive qualities are to be implanted.

The inner struggle is really the battle of Mahabharata, and it is an eternal one. This inward struggle is the price we must pay for the eternal reward of liberation. The winner ultimately is going to be Arjuna, who has made Lord Krishna as his charioteer.

BELIEF SYSTEM

Understanding beliefs and learning how to eliminate

negative ones and inculcate positive ones is like learning to operate the ruder of our life. As these beliefs are formed early in life, we take them as absolute truths and hardly dare to challenge them. As and when these beliefs are formed they seem logical at that time and useful also. We can hardly foresee that these very beliefs are going to limit our lives in future and create obstacles for us.

There are three words:

(1) Opinion
(2) Belief
(3) Conviction.

Opinion

There are three parameters which clarify opinion:

(a) It is a generalization.
(b) It is easily changeable.
(c) New information is interpreted independently of the opinion already held.

Belief

It is also a generalization, not easily changeable and new information is interpreted according to the already held belief.

Conviction

It is again a generalization, not changeable and no new information about it is entertained.

There are different layers of our personality at which we operate. If we count from outside to inside, these are environment, behaviour, capabilities. Beliefs, identity and spiritual. The deeper we are dealing with, the more pervasive and powerful it is and is capable of changing those superficial to it. Norman Cousins, the author of "The anatomy of an illness" writes, "Belief can create Biology."

Power of Belief

The power of belief is limitless. The placebo effect is an example of the power of belief. In double blind studies carried out for the effectiveness of drugs up to 30% of the people get well who believe that they are getting the proper treatment of their disease from the doctors although in reality they are only receiving glucose powder or any other such innocuous material. There are innumerable examples in medical literature where healing of so-called incurable diseases has occurred. Instead of studying such healings we have labeled them as spontaneous cures and left it at that. Even if we can achieve 30% cure rate in diseases, which at present moment labeled as incurable by modern medicine by changing the beliefs of the persons, it can be a worthy achievement. Robert Dilts changed the beliefs of her mother who was suffering from metastasized breast carcinoma, who became healed without the need of radiation, chemotherapy or any other conventional treatment. Seven years follow-up revealed no cancer symptoms. Dr. Bernie Segal's book "Love medicine and miracles" is full of instances of patients who participated in their healing by change of beliefs, visualization, etc. besides the conventional treatment of the doctors. Dr. Dean Ornish achieved a cure rate of 92% in coronary artery disease patients by changing their beliefs about themselves, others around them and about God, along with diet and exercise. Dr. Ornish showed that the blocked arteries of the patients actually started opening up which was demonstrated first time in the history of modern medicine.

Types of Beliefs

Beliefs can be divided in many ways:

(A) There are two types of beliefs:

(1) Positive or empowering beliefs; and
(2) Negative or disempowering or limiting beliefs.

Positive beliefs are those which make us more confident, competent and happy while negative ones decrease our confidence, competence and happiness.

(B) Another way to distinguish beliefs is:

(1) Global, and
(2) Local.

Global beliefs are those which operate in many areas of our lives, for example, a person can belief "Other people are out there to rip you apart if you give them a chance." Such a belief will come into play whenever we are dealing with other people. Local beliefs are applicable in only one area of our lives, e.g. "I am poor in maths."

(C) Types of beliefs according to origin: Beliefs about cause you can have beliefs about what causes something What causes cancer? What causes a person to be creative? What makes your business successful? What causes you to smoke? What causes you to fail at losing weight? The answer you give will be a statement of belief.

You might say, "If I go out without a coat in winter outside I will catch a cold. "The word because (actual or implied) often indicates a belief about a cause. A patient coming with vomiting and diarrohrea believes that this is caused by "bhai" created by eating rice and curry and by the infected food eaten 24 to 48 hours earlier. Subseqûent action will depend upon what belief he continues to hold. Beliefs about cause come from filters of your experience. If you believe that "x" causes something your behaviour will be directed towards making "X" happen or stopping it from happening if it has negative consequences.

Beliefs about Meaning

You can have beliefs about meaning. What do events mean or what is important or necessary? What does it mean to have cancer? If you have cancer does that mean you are a bad person and are being punished? Does it mean that you are out to kill yourself? Does it mean that you mean that you need to make changes in your lifestyle? What does it mean if you cannot quit smoking? Does it mean that you are weak? Does it mean that you are a failure? Does it mean that you have not integrated two parts yet?

Beliefs about meaning will result in behaviours congruent with the belief. If you believe that your difficulty in quitting smoking has to do with two unintegrated parts, you will probably work towards integrating them. If you believe that it means you are weak, you may not take action towards integration.

Beliefs about Identity

Beliefs about identity include cause, meaning and boundaries. What causes you to do something? What do your behaviours mean? What are your personal limits and boundaries? When you change your beliefs about your identity it mean you are going to be a different person somehow. Examples of limiting beliefs of identity are: "I am worthless", "I do not deserve to succeed" or "If I get what I want I will lose something." Beliefs about identity are also the beliefs that may keep you from changing, especially because you are often not conscious of them.

Sources of Beliefs

There are four different sources from which beliefs are formed.

Personal Experiences and the Meaning drawn out of those

Our most firm beliefs are formed from the experiences we undergo and the meanings we extract out of these experiences. Different people form different meaning out of similar experiences, e.g. two people is rejected in an interview for a job. One of them feels that some kind of push in the form of money or connections is required for getting the job while the other person thinks that he has poor technical knowledge which needs to be improved for getting the job. The first person will focus on finding the right connection while the second one will focus on upgrading his technical skill.

Experience of others

Experiences of significant other people in our lives are also passed on to us as our beliefs. Our parents, relatives, teachers, friends and other significant persons in our lives pass on their experiences to us and many times we corporate them in our belief system.

Role of Media

Many of our beliefs are created by media like television newspapers, radio, magazines, films, etc. Advertisements in the media bombard us daily with sponsored information and we form beliefs out of that.

Imagination

Some of our beliefs are also formed by our imagination. Many times we attribute something to other people in our imagination and firmly believe in it

How Beliefs are Formed

All the beliefs start as ideas. An idea can be considered like a table top. It cannot stand of its own. Suppose a person gets cold. He reviews the events of the recent past. His minds picks up any unusual event happening in the recent past and connects the two, e.g. a patient believes that whenever she takes a cold drink she gets an attack of asthma. The first time she got an attack of breathlessness, she asked herself inside, "What it could be due to." She picked up the non-routine event from her recent past, i.e. taking a cold drink. The meaning she drew out of that was probably cold drink does not suit me. From then on every time she got an attack of breathlessness, this idea flashed back in her mind and she associated cold drink with asthma till it got so firmly entrenched that her mind started directed the body accordingly.

Identifying Beliefs

Beliefs are often hard to define for a person. These might typically have to do with what can or cannot do, should or should not do, or ought or ought not to do. You might also hear, "I am this way", "I am a poor speller", I am a fat person. These statements indicate identity beliefs that limit the person's thinking about themselves, and what they can do to change.

Beliefs may also be stated as cause-effect phenomena, that are often stated in "If/then" kinds of statements. "If I do not say my prayers, I will be punished." "If I assert myself, then I will get rejected." "Just when I start to succeed, everything turns to garbage."

Finally, beliefs can often be identified by finding a problem situation, the person has unsuccessfully tried to change using a variety of methods. When you ask what does it mean about you that you have not been able to change this? you sometimes get an identity belief statement in response.

Pitfalls in Identifying Beliefs

(1) One of the problems, then in identifying beliefs is that you as a helper, tend to find substantiation for your beliefs in someone else.

(2) When persons tell about beliefs you will often get logical constructs to make sense out of certain behaviour they engage in. Many persons will change their free floating anxiety into such logical statements. Actually these feelings emanate from internal conflicts.

(3) In trying to identify beliefs of identity or a painful issue, a person might start blanking out or become confused and start discussing something very different.

CHANGING NEGATIVE BELIEFS INTO POSITIVE

Belief strategies are highly patterned and they can last a lifetime. This is fortunate, because without these strategies, our understanding of ourselves and the world would not be stable.

The belief strategies work as automatically and as durability for limiting beliefs as they do for beliefs that propel us toward our potential. Luckily they have a definite structure that can be elicited, so they can also be changed at the most basic levels if thinking through conscious intervention.

Step 1. Identify the negative belief.

Step 2. Create an idea, which is opposite to negative belief.

Step 3. Visualize experiences from your life, which strengthen the new idea and automatically weaken the old negative belief. There are bound to be many such experiences as belief is a generalization and every generalization has exceptions.

Step 4. Attach pain with the old negative belief. Visualize all negative consequences, which can happen if you continue to believe in the negative belief.

Step 5. Attach pleasure with the new idea. Visualize all pleasant experiences which are possible if we change to new idea/belief.

Step 6. From now on interpret the events according to the new idea consciously for three weeks till it becomes automatic.

Beliefs can also be charged by NLP. (Neurolinguistic programming)

DIFFERENT TECHNIQUES FOR DIFFERENT DISEASES

As different diseases require different treatment modalities, similarly different patients with the same disease or different diseases will require modified instructions as per the subjective experiences of the individual. Specific visualizations are required for different individuals and diseases. Basic processes are:

(1) Know what you want. Use affirmations or other techniques to deal with any internal objections to having what you want.
(2) Get into a relaxed, receptive state of mind.
(3) Visualize having or seeing what you want in as rich a way as possible.
(4) Expect and believe, you will receive it.
(5) Tell yourself that you deserve it.

People who have difficulty making visualizations work are often seeing a dissociated image of themselves doing what they want or having their outcome. Sometimes it is even a small framed still picture that is anything but compelling. On the other hand, successful visualizers are able to see a fully associated experience of having achieved their outcome. This means they are seeing what they want through their own eyes, as well as hearing, touching, moving, smelling and tasting their outcome, as if it were happening in their present experience. This kind of visualization results in a positive feeling and reinforces practice of the technique.

Response expectancy, the belief that something will

happen as the result of the action, is also important. Those who are successful experience their outcome in the visual, auditory and kinesthetic sub-modalities of expectations.

To create your own sub-modalities of expectancy, think of something you always do, such as sleep at night. Check how you think about that. What internal pictures are you making? Are you saying something to yourself or hearing other sounds. What kinesthetics are involved—feelings of movement or touch.

The non-successful visualizers often code their internal experience in the sub-modalities of hope or even doubt. To check the sub-modalities of hope, think of something you hope will happen. You will like it to happen, but do not know for sure that it will—such as getting a promotion at work. Examine your internal pictures, sounds and kinesthetics. The most common kinds of sub-modalities include fuzzy pictures, dissociated movies, a questioning tonality of voice, or multiple representations (pictures of having something and pictures of not having it that are flashing back and forth or that are seen at the same time.)

If when using the visualization process for health, you include a well formed outcome, a fully associated experience of already having the outcome, plus the sub-modalities of expectations, chances are that you will be more successful in achieving your goal.

FORMULA FOR BEHAVIOURAL CHANGE

(1) Decide what you truly want. It must be something that is within your control and something you do want, not "do not want." Determine how will you know when you have achieved your outcome. What will you see, hear and feel that will provide evidence?

+

What are the positive and negative consequences of getting your outcome? Modify your outcome to take care of any internal or external negative consequences.

Deal with any reservations you may have about getting your outcome. Write down reasons why you can't have it, allow yourself to fully experience any negative feelings that you might have, and create affirmation (positive self-statement) to release any blocks you might be experiencing.)

(2) Get into a receptive state of mind.

(3) Think of something that you fully and without reservation expect to happen. Go inside yourself and notice the qualities of your internal pictures (sub-modalities: colour, location, brightness, clarity, number of pictures), your sounds and voices (Tonal qualities, volume, pitch) and your feelings (tactile senses, sense of motion, action sense) for expecting that something will happen. Write these qualities down to keep track of them.

(4) Fully imagine seeing yourself having achieved your outcome as if you were watching a movie of yourself.

+

If you don't like the way it looks, modify it until you do.

+

If it looks "right" and you have no reservations about it, step into your movie and imagine that you are now experiencing having your outcome, using the sub-modalities of expectation.

(5) Let it go tell yourself that you deserve it.

METAPHOR—ORGAN LANGUAGE AND IDIOMS

The s/c mind often understands the language literally and the organ language statements might help as a diagnostic tool.

Skin Problems

Rash decision, itching to get on to something, scratch for a living.

Ulcer, Stomach Problems

Something eating you? Sick to the stomach, something you can't stomach, to do something takes lot of guts.

Headaches, Neck Problems

Somebody or something pain in the neck, head on into some problems, weight on your shoulders

Weight Problems; Weighty Problems

Eyesight; Don't want to look at something, dim view of something, nothing is clear.

Constipation

Holding something back, tight rein on things, hold on to your problems, things never go smoothly.

Heart

Breaking the heart, experiencing heartache, doing things half-heartedly.

CREATING SUPPORT GROUPS

If these measures can be introduced in larger hospitals on a regular basis then support groups can be created where persons already recovered from similar problems can guide persons who are in the process of making that recovery. Such mutual support plays a very important role in life threatening problems and may be a crucial factor in tilting the balance in favour of health.

CREATING TANGIBLE TARGETS

In Second World War about ten percent of persons survived the life of concentration camps. A doctor who himself survived conducted a survey about the characteristics of people who came alive out of such camps. He found out that all of them have one common thing and that is all of them have something tangible to live for. Their goals were not some lofty spiritual attainments but much more concrete and worldly ones like publishing a book, or asking pardon from somebody before dying, or meeting an offspring born after their confinement in concentration camp. If we can create such goals for persons from life threatening problems, they can turn their unutilized hidden resources for survival and healing. Therefore, goal setting is another area to be discussed with them.

Characteristics of Goals

There are four main characteristics:

1. Excitability,
2. High,
3. Specific, and
4. Self-defendant

Areas in which Goals are to be Created

(1) Personal development goals.
(2) Economic goals.
(3) Entertainment goals.
(4) Contributory goals.

If we can create such departments where every person from life threatening problems undergoes these self-development experiences and contributes and participates in his or her own healing, healthy living and peaceful dying can become more common. Creating such departments will hardly take large financial investments and rapport between the doctors and the patients can create synergetic healing. Besides the above mentioned methods, physical exercise and diet also play an important part in the healing process.

GUIDELINES FOR PATIENTS SUFFERING FROM LIFE THREATENING PROBLEMS

1. Patient should decide to spend two to three hours with himself for learning and carrying out different techniques of healing.
2. He should explore various treatment options available to him and decide about the modality of

treatment after consulting different specialists.

3. Once he has decided about it, he should enter the treatment with total belief about its effectiveness.
4. He should start learning about the disease as to how it occurs and spreads and how it can be cured. He should not bother about the statistics about survival nor should allow his doctor to predict his longevity. The statistics do not apply to individual patients.
5. He should start taking one hour of walk with a speed which does not make him breathless.
6. He should start learning and performing about ten to fifteen yogic asanas.
7. He should start learning and performing about four to five pranayama exercises.
8. He should learn and practice directed and receptive visualization.

The patient should learn and start developing more intimate relationships with others around him by expressing his feelings and not thoughts, with the help of compassion, altruism, appreciation and non-judgemental attitude.

He should learn the art and practice of meditation on a regular basis.

He is to learn to form positive beliefs about himself and others and throw out the negative ones.

These techniques mentioned above lead to intimacy with oneself, intimacy with a higher self and intimacy with others. Experience of isolation is the most important factor in the causation of disease.

13

Let Your Vision be Clear: Remove Cobwebs of Eye Myths

R.K. GREWAL*

Alongwith great grandmother's ornaments and family photographs, myths about health are passed from one generation to the next, and ideas about eye care are no exception. But it is important to distinguish between fact and fiction. Knowledge about eye care is the first step to protecting your sight for a lifetime.

COMMON EYE MYTHS

Eating Carrots will Improve your Vision

It is true that carrots are high in Vitamin A, which is necessary for the development of normal vision (which is usually complete by age six). There is no evidence that overdoing it will improve vision. However, only a small amount is required a good diet with or without carrots, provides plenty of Vitamin A.

* Professor and Head, Dept. of Ophthalmology, Dayanand Medical College and Hospital Ludhiana.

Reading in Dim Light can Damage your Eyes

Reading in dim light does not affect vision but the effort required can cause eye fatigue, but will not worsen any refractory error. However, for comfort, the reading material should be adequately illuminated either by daylight or by adequate positioning of the light source.

Excessive Reading, Sewing or doing other Close Work Decreases Vision

For hundreds of years, reading or sewing at night was done by candlelight, or with gas or kerosene lamps. Good lighting and right glasses make things more comfortable and less stressful but their absence does not decrease vision.

People with 'Weak Eyes' should Avoid Reading Fine Print"

It is a common belief that people who wear glasses have weak eyes and will further harm their eyes if they read fine print or do a lot of detail work. The eyes do not get any sort of damage by reading fine print. Again, adequate comfort should be provided.

Excessive Crying especially due to Bereavement Causes Decreased Vision

Excessive tear formation as in crying is a response to emotion and has no effect on vision. If there is decreased vision, it should never be attributed to excessive crying.

Looking at the Solar Eclipse is a Good Omen

It is believed to be a good omen by our elders but they always looked at it through reflection from water. Normally, the sun is too bright and on looking at it, the discomfort makes us turn our eyes away and our pupils constrict preventing excessive rays from entering the eye. While watching a solar eclipse off a little, a flood of light and heat enter through our dilated pupils, and cause damage to the retina causing visual loss. Therefore, we should never watch a solar eclipse with naked eyes. Special filters or better still a projection on the wall using a pin hole camera should be used.

Failure to use Proper Glasses will Worsen Nearsightedness

Nearsightedness is a hereditary condition in which the eye length becomes longer than normal so that a distant object is not focused on the retina. This myopia increases as the child grows usually upto the age of adolescence irrespective of him using the glasses or not. Therefore myopic children should get their eyes checked every year.

Eye Exercises can Remove Glasses

Eye exercises can alleviate eye strain due to muscle imbalance. Only any refractive error can only be corrected by glasses or contact lenses.

Contact Lenses can Prevent Nearsightedness and Myopia from getting Worse

Some people think wearing contact lenses will permanently correct nearsightedness and myopia, and eventually they might be able to get rid of their glasses or contact lenses. Contact lenses improve refractory errors while you are wearing them just as glasses do, but do not reverse the condition or keep it from becoming worse. Myopia progresses up to adolescence after which it stabilizes. So, yearly refraction should be done.

Contact Lenses can Slip Back and become Lost behind the Eye"

The contact lens can only slip into the fornices and can easily be removed. The thin tissue connecting the eyelid to the back of the eye prevents the lens from going further back.

Contact Lens Wear Decreases the Power of your Prescription

It is not true the contact lenses can in any way decrease the power of correction required. They correct the vision just like glasses

Sitting too Long/too Close to the Television or Holding a Book too Close to your Eyes is the Cause of Children Wearing Glasses

Children can focus up close without eyestrain better

than adults can. Some children develop the habit of sitting too close to the television or holding a book too close. There is no evidence this practice will decrease their vision, and the habit usually disappears as the child grows older. However, children who have poor distant vision will also tend to sit closer to the TV or hold a book too close. Therefore, this may be an early sign and not the cause of decreased vision. Such children should have their eyes tested for any refractive error.

Using Computers can Damage your Eyes

Working on the computer does not contribute in any way towards refractive errors. You can develop eye fatigue, strain or a dry eye after looking at one for long periods of time, just as you can from reading or doing other close work. To relieve eye strain, take regular breaks and look up or across the room. Looking at objects further away usually relieves eyestrain. While working on the computer, the blink rate decreases which may cause dry eyes and discomfort. Therefore, one must remember to blink more often while on computer.

With Age, Squint Disappears

Children don't outgrow squint with age. A child with misaligned eyes may develop amblyopia (lazy eye), in which the brain ignores input from the squinting eye resulting in further loss of vision. We need to treat the amblyopia while the brain is still developing the visual system, preferably upto the age 6. One strategy is to patch the stronger eye to stimulate the weaker eye. As a rule the younger the child presenting for treatment, the better the outcome.

An Eye Examination is Necessary only if you're having Problems

This is not true. Children should have an eye and vision examination before 5 years of age. Early detection and treatment of childhood eye conditions such as squint and amblyopia can help ensure a lifetime of good vision. Eye problems such as glaucoma (which is rightly called the sneak thief of sight), usually have no symptoms in the early stages of the disease, and if left untreated, can cause permanent vision loss. Other systemic diseases like diabetes and hypertension are silent killers and when detected late cannot retrieve the damage already done. Hence, a thorough eye examination every two years should be mandatory for people above 45 years of age.

Conjunctivitis Spreads through Air

It is a contagious disease but can be spread through contact like using common linen, soap or by handshake. By merely looking at the eyes of an infected patient, one cannot get conjunctivitis.

Cataract can be Prevented or Reversed by Eye Drops

Most common type of cataract is related to aging. In some, it occurs earlier than others but there is no evidence that any medication can prevent the occurrence of cataract or reverse it. Please see Appendix V, Free Radicals and antioxidants for latest trends in prevention of cataract and other eye ailments.

Cataracts have to "ripen" before they are Removed

Unlike the old days, cataract surgery can now be done at any stage. The latest techniques get rid of the cataract irrespective of the status of maturity.

It is totally patient dependent and should be removed when the visual loss interferes with your everyday activities, such as reading, driving, watching TV. You and your eye doctor should make this decision together. Waiting until you are ready to have cataract surgery will not harm your eye.

Oily and Spicy Food after Cataract Removal can affect the Eyes

After cataract surgery, there are no restrictions, neither on your food nor in your movements. You can lead a normal life just as before from day one.

IOL is the Cure for All

IOL is an artificial lens, which replaces the cataractous lens on removal and thereby helps to focus the objects on the retina. It does not improve vision when the cornea or the retina is damaged.

Cataract Surgery is done with a Laser

Cataract surgery is not performed using lasers. It is a surgery in which the lens is converted into a gel form by an ultrasonic device and then aspirated. In other words, it still remains to be a surgery. Sometimes the patient develops a translucent opacity leading to decrease in vision for which we can make a small pin hole in the center using a laser.

Decreased Vision in Old Age is only because of Cataract

Decreased vision in old age can be due to innumerable causes including presbyopia which is correctable by glasses alone, hypermetropia, some systemic disease and many other ailments.

Surgery gets rid of Glaucoma for ever

The vernacular name for glaucoma "kala motia" makes people believe that like cataract "chita motia", it can totally be cured once surgery is done. Glaucoma, in fact is like hypertension. It is only controlled as long as you are on medication or it is under the control after surgery. In spite of being controlled today, it may become uncontrolled later on without any symptoms and do the irreversible damage. So, once you have glaucoma, a monitoring as to the pressure of eye, retinal examination and visual field recording has to continue periodically throughout one's life and whenever the doctor feels the need, he will make alterations to the modality of treatment. So glaucoma surgery is not the final word in a glaucoma patient.

Eyes can be Transplanted

The eye is connected to the brain by the optic nerve (made up of millions of nerve fibers), which cannot be reconnected once it is severed. Hence, there is no way to transplant the whole eye. The eye is never removed from its socket during surgery. Only the cornea, the clear front part of the eye, can be transplanted for conditions where it becomes opaque.

All 'Eye Doctors' are the Same

An ophthalmologist is a doctor who specializes in the

eye and its diseases and can provide all facets of eye care including surgery. Optometrists/opticians are basically technicians for only assisting in refractions and can in no way diagnose/treat other causes of visual loss. Many of them take on to practice, which is ideally called quackery. Therefore, once you have problems with vision, you must have an ophthalmologist check your eyes to ascertain the cause of decrease in vision.

Girls with Blue Eyes are Unreliable

Surely untrue. If it were so, Aishwarya Rai would not have been the most sought after woman on earth.

14

Breast Feeding is the Best: Save it from Cancer

GURPREET SINGH*

Breast feeding is considered good for the child as well as mother. Mother should not deny this gift of nature to her new born, at least in the first 6-12 months of his/her life. It provides nutrition, immune bodies and a feeling of love and affection for the child and satisfaction for the mother. While the importance of this organ cannot be over emphasized, the incidence of its ailments, esp. breast cancer is also rising fast. Certain preventive measures can help to preserve this organ of feminine pride and nutrition.

What is Breast Cancer?

Breast cancer is a potentially life-threatening cancer that develops in one or both breasts. Breast cancer is either **non-invasive** (confined to the site of origin) or **invasive** (spreading to other sites in the body). Before we proceed further let us see what cancer is? Through the natural cycle of life, cells divide to create new tissue as older cells die-off. When tissue is injured, for instance by a cut on the hand, the body's cell growth regulators react by speeding up the process of cell division to create new tissue in the injured area as fast as possible. When the body has healed, the creation of new tissue through cell division goes back to the normal pace. In a healthy body, there are natural mechanisms

* Professor, Department of Surgery, Postgraduate Institute of Medical Education and Research, Chandigarh.

that regulate the creation, growth, and death of cells. Cancer is a disease where the natural regulators malfunction and cells do not die off at the right rate. As a result, cell growth goes haywire. Cancer cells divide without control, accumulating into a mass of extra tissue—a **tumor**. Cancer cells can also leave the tumor site and travel through the blood stream and lymphatic system (the network connecting lymph nodes throughout the body) to other parts of the body, such as the liver, lungs, or bones. This process of cancer cells leaving the original tumor and appearing elsewhere is called **metastasis**. In the new location, cancer cells will again begin to divide abnormally to create a tumor. A person with cancer will eventually die of the disease when vital organs like the liver or lungs are invaded and destroyed.

Non-invasive Breast Cancers

Ductal carcinoma in situ **(DCIS)**: DCIS consist of cancer cells in the lining of the duct. DCIS is a non-invasive, early cancer, but if left untreated, it may sometimes progress to an invasive, infiltrating ductal breast cancer.

Lobular carcinoma in situ **(LCIS)**: Although non-invasive, lobular carcinoma *in situ* is a marker for an increased risk of invasive cancer in both breasts. Patients with LCIS run the risk of developing invasive cancer in the same breast in about 18% and in the other breast in 14% after 20 years.

Invasive Breast Cancer

When cancer cells spread beyond the *cell of origin*, the tumor becomes invasive. The surrounding tissue is rich in blood vessels and lymphatic channels that are capable of carrying cancer cells beyond the breast. Invasive breast cancers include the following:

Infiltrating ductal carcinoma: This is invasive breast cancer that penetrates the wall of a duct. It comprises between 70% and 80% of all breast cancer cases.

Infiltrating lobular carcinoma: This invasive cancer has spread through the wall of a lobule. It accounts for between 10% and 15% of all breast cancers. It may sometimes appear in both breasts, sometimes in several separate locations. There are other less common invasive breast cancers.

What Is 'Risk' and What are Risk Factors for Developing Breast Cancer

Risk is a person's chance of developing a specific disease over a specified time period. It is commonly noted that the lifetime risk of breast cancer for an American woman born in 1990 is about 1 in 8, if she lives to be 85. This means that for every 8 women who live to be age 85, one of them will have been diagnosed with breast cancer during her lifetime. A risk factor can be anything from a lifestyle choice (such as diet) to genetic make-up to an environmental exposure (such as radiation) that increases a person's risk of developing a certain disease. Often, when the news media present new research findings on breast cancer, they do not give information on absolute risk. Instead, information is provided in terms of the increase in risk due to a particular risk factor. It is critical to recognize that the importance of a relative risk depends on the underlying absolute risks. For example, if a person has a single rupee, this makes rupees "rare." If this person doubles her money, she only gains an extra rupee. In contrast, if a person has a million rupees, this makes rupees "common," and a doubling of her money means she gains a million extra rupees. In both cases, there is a doubling of money, but the real increase in rupees is very different.

Risk Factors that cannot be Controlled

Age is a well-established risk factor for breast cancer. The older a woman is, the more likely she is to develop the disease. In general, rates of breast cancer are low in women under age 40, begin to increase after age 40, and are highest in women over age 70.

Family history is an important factor contributing to a woman's chance of developing breast cancer. Having an immediate family member (mother, sister, daughter) with breast cancer increases a woman's chance of developing breast cancer 2 to 3 times compared to a woman with no family history of the disease. If a woman has a history of more than one immediate family member with breast cancer, her chance is increased by about 4 times compared to a woman with no family history. In general, the younger her relative was when diagnosed with breast cancer, the greater a woman's chance of getting the disease. While family history of breast cancer can be due to many factors (such as family lifestyle), it can also be associated with specific genetic changes (mutations) that can increase susceptibility for the disease. This is especially so in families with a strong family history of breast cancer, such as multiple immediate family members with breast cancer or a single immediate family member diagnosed at an early age.

Having been diagnosed with **breast cancer previously** is a strong risk factor for developing breast cancer again in the other breast. The new cancer that develops is called a second primary breast cancer. The risk of developing a second breast cancer in women with previous breast cancer is about 0.5 to 1.0 percent per year.

LCIS is considered to be a risk factor for the development of invasive cancer, rather than a condition that develops into invasive disease. Compared to women without LCIS, those with the condition have about a 7 to 10-fold increase in the risk of developing cancer in either breast.

The term **benign breast disease** has traditionally been used to describe a wide range of non-cancerous breast disorders, some of which increase the risk of breast cancer and some of which do not. Proliferative breast disease increases the risk of breast cancer and refers to non-cancerous disorders characterized by multiplying (proliferating) cells.

Risk Factors that can be Controlled

While a woman's family history and genetic make-up cannot be controlled, there are certain risk factors that can be modified in an attempt to reduce the risk of developing breast cancer. Although some of these factors—particularly the reproductive ones—can be hard to modify because of social norms and cultural demands, many are more readily modifiable and are important parts of an overall healthy lifestyle.

The hormone **estrogen** plays an important role in

breast cancer. A high cumulative lifetime exposure to estrogen—primarily through the hormones released by ovaries during the menstrual cycle—also appears to increase the risk of breast cancer. A woman's **age at menarche** and her **age at menopause** can indicate how many years she was exposed to the higher estrogen levels associated with menstrual cycles. Exposure to estrogen may seem like it is totally out of a woman's control, but there are a number of lifestyle factors that can play a role in increasing a woman's exposure to the hormone. These factors include such things as being overweight after menopause, drinking alcohol, being physically inactive and currently or recently using post-menopausal hormones.

A large analysis that combined the results of numerous studies found that women who were currently taking or recently took **oral contraceptives** had a 10 to 30 percent higher risk of breast cancer than women who had never used birth control pills. The good news, though, was that this increased risk began to diminish as soon as the women stopped taking oral contraceptives, and disappeared after about ten years.

Women who have **never given birth** or who do so for the **first time after the age of 30** have a higher risk of breast cancer than women who give birth before age 30. For women who have their first child after the age of 30, the risk of breast cancer increases two-fold when compared with women who have their first child before the age of 20. In addition to age at first having a child, the number of children that a woman has in her lifetime also has a small effect on her risk of breast cancer.

Healthy Behaviours and the Risk of Breast Cancer

Although there is no sure way for a woman to prevent breast cancer, enough information exists about known risk factors that women can take steps that may modify their risk of developing the disease. The most important thing for women to remember is that healthy behaviours that may decrease the risk of breast cancer may also lower the risk of many other major chronic diseases, such as heart disease, diabetes, colon cancer and osteoporosis. Therefore, the following is a list of things women can do to improve their overall health:

- Be physically active.
- Maintain a healthy weight.
- Eat a diet that is rich in fruits, vegetables and whole grains and that emphasizes good fats (monounsaturated and polyunsaturated fats) over bad fats (saturated and trans fats).
- Take a daily multivitamin.
- Limit alcohol intake.
- Choose to breastfeed children instead of formula feeding them.

Genes and Breast Cancer Risk

A number of genes have been linked to breast cancer, including BRCA1, BRCA2 (standing for Breast Cancer gene 1 and 2). While mutations in these genes have been shown to greatly increase the chances of developing breast cancer, not all women with such mutations develop the disease. Moreover, only 5 to 10 percent of all breast cancers can be attributed to inherited genetic mutations that have already been identified. Women who carry a BRCA1 mutation are thought to have a 60 to 80 percent chance of developing breast cancer in their lifetimes. Women with a BRCA2 mutation appear to have a slightly lower lifetime risk—about 30 to 80 percent. However, it is important to remember that most breast cancer is not hereditary or genetic. And, even in the case of BRCA mutations, genes do not seem to equal destiny. About 20 to 40 percent of women with a BRCA1 mutation do not develop breast cancer, so it is likely that a combination of factors ultimately determines who will develop the disease. These mutations can be passed down to the daughter by either the mother or the father.

Genetic testing provides individuals the opportunity to determine if their family history of breast cancer may be due to a BRCA1 or BRCA2 mutation. Because the mutations greatly increase risk, having the knowledge of one's genetic status can allow an individual to take certain steps to try to prevent the onset of breast cancer or to diagnose and treat it in early stages when it is most curable. Although the tests for the BRCA1 and 2 mutations require only a blood sample, there are many risks and benefits that should be weighed in depth before an individual goes through with the testing.

Risks

- Adverse psychological impact of knowing results.
- Negative test does not mean absence of other inherited risks.
- Negative test does not mean that the person will not get breast cancer.

Benefits

- Knowledge of genetic status for self and family members.
- Opportunity to plan life based on test results.
- Opportunity to take an option for risk reduction.

Options for Women at High Risk for Breast Cancer

Close surveillance refers to an increase in screening frequency for high-risk patients.

Bilateral prophylactic mastectomy is the removal of both breasts in an attempt to keep cancer from developing in the first place. Prophylactic bilateral mastectomy can lower the risk of breast cancer in high-risk women by up to 90 percent. Prophylactic mastectomy does not completely protect a woman from breast cancer.

Chemoprevention refers to the use of drugs to reduce the risk of breast cancer. Tamoxifen is the most well studied chemoprevention drug to date. Tamoxifen lowers the chances of developing invasive breast cancer by about 49 percent. The FDA (USA) has approved the use of tamoxifen to reduce the incidence of breast cancer in high-risk women.

Early Detection

Getting regular breast cancer screening tests is the single best way to lower the risk of dying from breast cancer. By finding the disease early, before any symptoms arise, these tests greatly improve the chances of successful treatment. There are three standard screening techniques currently available to women: **mammography, clinical breast examination,** and **breast self-examination (BSE).** Although a few scientific controversies still exist in the field of breast cancer screening, there is general consensus that appropriate, regular screening saves lives.

The quality of a screening test is described in terms of its accuracy in telling who truly has an illness (its sensitivity) and who does not (its specificity). Simply put, the primary goal of a screening test is to make sure that every person who is tested and has the disease is identified as having it (100% sensitivity). Likewise, an ideal screening test would also be able to identify all the people who do not have the disease as not having it (100% specificity). A perfect test then would be able to identify everyone accurately with no mix-ups. Mammography and clinical breast exam are each reasonably sensitive, but their sensitivity improves when they are used in combination. With mammography alone, about 15 to 20 percent of cases may be missed, but with both mammography and clinical breast exam included in a woman's annual check-up, the chances of a tumor going undetected are cut down to less than 5 percent.

Mammography is a technique using X-rays to find breast lumps that cannot be felt either because they are too small or because they have an indistinct shape. During the procedure, which usually takes about 15 minutes, each breast is compressed between two plates, and an X-ray image is made. Overall, mammography is the best screening tool available today. However, mammograms may be more effective at detecting tumors in older women than in younger women, and some debate still exists about the exact benefits of mammograms in younger women.

Women Ages 50-69: There is no debate about the life-saving importance of mammography in this age group: all women between the ages of 50 and 69 should receive an annual mammogram. This recommendation is based on scientific evidence that has been accumulating since the 1960s from randomized controlled trials conducted in the United States, Canada and Europe. In these trials, women who were screened annually with mammography had a 25 to 30 percent lower risk of dying from breast cancer than their peers who were not screened annually.

Women Ages 40-49: A number of randomized controlled trials have shown that mammography in women ages 40 to 49 can lower the risk of dying from breast cancer. However, some debate still remains about the exact magnitude and timing of this benefit. The reason that mammography might be less beneficial in younger women than in older women is not yet clear.

Clinical Breast Examination is a physical examination done by physicians, nurses, and other trained medical staff. Checking the feel and look of the breasts for signs of lumps, a medical professional examines the breasts when the woman is sitting upright and while lying down. Although often overshadowed by the promotion of regular mammograms, clinical breast examinations are an important part of breast cancer screening. Not only has clinical breast examination been shown to be just as accurate as mammography, but it has also been suggested that for younger women, clinical breast examination may have an advantage over mammography. Clinical breast examinations are generally started much earlier than mammograms. Other benefit of clinical breast examination is that it can be done as part of a routine medical check-up and is comparatively inexpensive. In addition, the examiner can tell right away if he has found anything abnormal that will require follow-up testing.

Clinical breast exam and mammography should be thought of as complementary techniques, because regular screening with both will increase chances for early detection.

Breast Self-Examination is intended to increase a woman's chances of detecting a small tumor by herself. Of particular importance with breast self-examination is the opportunity to detect tumors that develop in the time between annual mammograms and clinical breast examination. By doing self-examination once a month, women can become familiar with the way their breasts look and feel normally and thus may be able to recognize changes such as thickening, lumps, or spontaneous nipple discharge (Figure 1).

FIG. I

Breast Self Examination: Technique

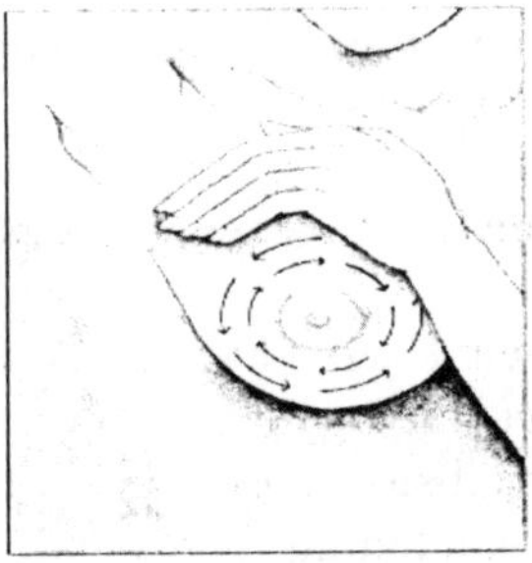

A: Stand in front of a mirror and look at each breast separately. Note the size, shape, colour, contour and direction of your breasts and nipples.

B: Raise your arms over your head and look at your breasts, as you turn slowly from side to side.

C: Press your hands on your hips and push your shoulders forward. Look at each breast separately.

D: Stand in front of a mirror and start BSE just below the collarbone.

E: Use the left hand for the right breast. Moisten the pads of your three middle fingertips with body lotion. Apply firm pressure and make small circles as you go back or forth (up or down, circular or spoke style) in a pattern covering all the breast area including the nipple. Extend the examination to the breast tissue in the underarm. Change your hand and repeat BSE on the opposite breast.

F: Lie down and raise one arm above your head. Examine your breasts as before, omitting the underarm.

Change your arm and repeat BSE on the opposite breast.

Breast tissue naturally has a bumpy texture and there is a great deal of individual variation. In most cases, this lumpiness is no cause to worry. If the lumpiness can be felt throughout the breast, then it is probably just the normal contours of the breast tissue. The kinds of lumps that are of concern are ones that are referred to as "dominant," meaning that they are firmer than the rest of the breast. Any time a woman discovers a lump that feels dominant, she should have it checked by a medical professional.

Intuitively, breast self-exam seems like an ideal method of early detection, because it is something all women can do on their own, and the cost of self-examination is much lower than that of annual mammography or physician visits for clinical breast examination. Unfortunately, it is still unclear whether breast self-examination is a useful way for the majority of women to detect early stage tumors and improve their chances for survival, and there has been some controversy about whether it should even be included in screening recommendations.

What Happens when a Screening Test Finds Something Abnormal

For most women who have a clinical breast exam or mammogram, the results will be good news, with the test finding no signs of disease. For some women, though, the test will turn up something abnormal. These women will need to have additional tests to determine whether they have cancer.

Is it Cancer? Diagnosis of Breast Cancer

The question "is it cancer?" can be very frightening to a woman and her family and friends. A diagnosis of cancer has huge physical, emotional and financial implications. Understanding the many issues that relate to diagnosis (such as the tests involved, their accuracy, and what the results mean) can help a woman take control of her situation and pick the best course of action for her.

Biopsy

Two general categories of biopsies are used to diagnose breast cancer. These are:

Needle biopsies, which include:

- *Fine needle aspiration*
- *Core needle biopsy*

Open biopsies, which include:

- *Excisional biopsy (including wire localization)*
- *Incisional biopsy*

Needle biopsies use a needle to remove tissue or cells from the breast. Open biopsies are surgical procedures that open the breast to remove tissue. Each method has advantages and disadvantages. The method used depends on a number of factors, such as the type of abnormality a woman has in her breast and the practice pattern of her physicians.

Fine needle aspiration cytology, also known as fine needle aspiration biopsy, uses a thinner needle than that used in core needle biopsy to remove a sample of cells, rather than tissue, from the abnormal area of the breast. The cells removed during FNA are then analyzed under the microscope by a cytopathologist. Because cytopathologists are not available in many hospitals, the need for their expertise to analyze the cells removed by FNA is an important limitation of the procedure.

Core needle biopsy is a method that uses a thin, hollow needle to remove samples of tissue from the breast. These tissue samples are then examined by a pathologist to see if they are cancerous. Core needle biopsy can be used for both palpable masses and non-palpable lesions. When a core needle biopsy is done for a non-palpable lesion, ultrasound or a special type of mammography (stereo-tactic mammography) is needed to accurately guide the needle to the suspicious area.

Unlike the needle biopsies that take samples from a particular area, **excisional biopsy** is a surgical procedure that removes the entire suspected area (plus some surrounding normal tissue) from the breast. It is sometimes also referred to as "lumpectomy." When doing an excisional biopsy on a non-palpable lesion, the surgeon needs a guide to identify the breast tissue that is to be removed. The radiologist provides this guide by inserting a very thin wire into the breast to the targeted area. The surgeon then uses the wire as a guide to find and remove the abnormal area. This procedure is called wire localization or needle localization.

In addition to examining the removed tissue for cancer, a variety of other tests can be done that are essential to planning a woman's treatment.

Tests for Prognostic and Predictive Factors

The purpose of these tests is to determine :

- The extent of the spread of disease in the woman.
- The treatment the woman needs.
- The prognosis (outcome) of the woman.

Only about six percent of women have distant metastases when they are first diagnosed with breast cancer. A woman who experiences symptoms such as shortness of breath, chronic cough, weight loss or bone pain may have distant metastases. Only after some specific tests can their presence be confirmed or ruled out. The three primary tests performed are a blood test to check for spread to the liver and/ or bones, bone scans to test for spread to the bone and X-ray/CT scans to test for spread to the chest, abdomen and liver.

Lymph Node Status

When cancer forms in the breast, one of the first places it may spread to is the lymph nodes under the armpit, known as the axillary lymph nodes. Cancer has the best prognosis when it remains within the breast (localized). Any time it spreads beyond the breast to the lymph nodes, the prognosis worsens. As the number of cancerous nodes increased, survival rates decrease. Node status is determined primarily in two ways. The first method is by palpation during a physical examination, where a doctor feels under the arm to determine if the nodes are enlarged. This method, though, while fast and convenient, is not very accurate. The second, and more accurate method is to examine the nodes directly after they have been removed from under the armpit. This is called an axillary dissection and is usually done during the surgery performed to remove the tumor from the breast.

Increasingly, physicians are recommending a new option to evaluate the axilla for cancer, called a **sentinel node biopsy**. This procedure involves the removal of just the sentinel node (defined as the first node filtering lymph fluid from the tumor site). During this procedure, a colored dye and/or radioactive-labeled tracer is injected into the breast near the tumor. The first lymph node to pick up the dye or tracer is the sentinel node. This node is removed and sent to a pathologist, who examines it to see if it contains cancer cells. Only if the sentinel node is found to be cancerous does the patient then go on to have the more invasive axillary dissection.

Tumor Size

Numerous studies have found that the larger a woman's tumor is, the more likely it is that she will have positive lymph nodes. Tumor size is directly related to prognosis and can be determined in a number of ways. It can be assessed during a physical examination by touch, through imaging with ultrasound or mammography, or, most accurately, by examining a tumor taken out during surgery. In general, the larger the tumor, the worse the prognosis

Tumor Grade

By looking under a microscope at tissue taken during a biopsy, the pathologist determines how closely the cancer cells resemble normal tissue. The more they look like normal tissue, the lower the tumor grade. The pathologist also looks to see how many of the cancer cells are in the process of dividing. If a large number of cells are dividing, it means that the tumor is likely to be growing fast and will be given a higher grade. Other things being equal, the higher the grade of a tumor, the worse a woman's prognosis.

Hormone Receptor Status

Estrogen and progesterone are naturally-occurring female hormones that some breast cancers need to grow. Tumors that have many sites to which these hormones attach are known as hormone receptor positive. Whether a tumor has estrogen or progesterone receptors is a very important predictor of whether the tumor will respond to hormonal treatments. A receptor-positive tumor often needs hormones to grow, and treatment that blocks the hormones from the tumor may stop its growth. The drug most often used in this type of treatment is tamoxifen, and it is very effective against receptor-positive cancers. The receptor status of a tumor is determined by tests done on tissue removed during a biopsy.

While hormone receptor status is a very important

predictor for hormonal treatment, it is also associated with chances of recurrence. Tumors without estrogen or progesterone receptors have a higher chance of recurrence than those that are estrogen or progesterone receptor-positive.

HER2/neu (erbB^2)

HER2/neu is a protein that appears in high numbers on the outside of the breast cancer cells of some patients. Tumors with high levels of HER2/neu have been linked to more aggressive breast cancer and possibly to resistance or enhanced sensitivity to certain types of chemotherapy and hormone therapy. Tumors that express HER2/neu are also effective targets for the biological therapy drug, trastuzumab (Herceptin).

Staging of Breast Cancer

After a diagnosis of cancer has been confirmed, the cancer is classified into a particular stage. The stage of the cancer helps determine what treatment is necessary and how curative this treatment may be. The earlier the stage at diagnosis, the better the prognosis.

A number of methods for classifying stage exist. Most widely used, though, is the TNM classification. TNM takes into account the size of the tumor (T), the number of cancerous lymph nodes (N), and whether or not the cancer has spread to other areas of the body (metastasis-M). The stage of a cancer is usually determined at two separate times. The first time is based on results from a physical examination and tests like mammography (known as **clinical staging**), and the second time is based on a direct examination of the lymph nodes and tumor removed during surgery (known as **pathologic staging**). It is usual to divide breast cancer in four stages (with further sub-stages according to the prognosis). For convenience it can be classified into—

- Early (stage I & II)—Usually curable.
- Locally advanced (stage III)—Potentially curable.
- Metastatic (stage IV)—Incurable.

Treating Breast Cancer

The goal of treating breast cancer is to get rid of the cancer from the body and prevent it from returning. This is usually done with a combination of surgery, radiation therapy, chemotherapy, and hormone therapy. Surgery and radiation therapy are called local treatments. They focus on getting rid of the cancer from a limited (local) area, such as the breast, chest wall and lymph nodes under the armpit (axillary nodes). Chemotherapy and hormone therapy make up what is called systemic therapy. In systemic therapy, the entire body is treated to get rid of any cancer cells that may have spread from the breast tumor to other areas of the body.

What exactly makes up a woman's treatment depends on many factors, such as her age, tumor stage and estrogen receptor status. Each treatment option has risks and benefits. The type of treatment a woman decides upon should be based on an understanding of these risks and benefits and how they relate to her own personal values and lifestyle.

Treatment of Early Breast Cancer—Stages I and II

Surgery

The goal of surgery is to completely remove the tumor from the breast and to remove a number of lymph nodes from under the armpit (axillary dissection). There are basically two types of surgery for breast cancer—**breast conserving surgery** and **mastectomy.**

Breast conserving surgery (also known as **lumpectomy** or wide excision) is being used more and more in the treatment of breast cancer. The procedure is called "breast conserving" because only part of the breast—the part containing and closely surrounding the cancer—is removed. This leaves much of the breast looking as normal as possible. When lumpectomy is done, radiotherapy to the breast is a must and forms an integral part of breast conservation. In comparison, a total mastectomy is a complete removal of the breast. In the past, total mastectomy was the favoured treatment because it was thought to be the best means of getting rid of all the cancer in the breast and chest area.

Many studies have consistently shown that breast conserving surgery, when used with radiation therapy, is just as effective as total mastectomy in treating early-stage breast cancer. Not all women with early stage breast cancer, however, are eligible for breast conserving surgery plus radiation. Axillary dissection is done both in mastectomy and breast conserving surgery. This can be omitted if the new procedure of sentinel node biopsy is adopted.

The primary benefits of breast conserving surgery are that the woman's breast is preserved, and she avoids the emotional and psychological impact of having an entire breast removed. The primary benefit of total mastectomy is that radiation therapy is often not needed. For women living in remote areas, this can be an especially important benefit, allowing them to potentially avoid both the radiation therapy (and its side effects) and the long daily trips to a radiation therapy facility.

About 15-20 percent of women develop lymphedema (swelling of the arm) some time after treatment for their breast cancer. The accumulation of fluid, which causes the arm to swell, is associated with the removal of the lymph nodes from the armpit. The degree of lymphedema depends upon the number of lymph nodes removed from the axilla and whether the patient receives radiotherapy. Because lymphedema can be triggered by an injury or infection to the arm, patients should take these precautions whenever possible.

Breast reconstruction can help restore the look and feel of the breast that was removed during total mastectomy. This can be completed during the total mastectomy surgery (immediate reconstruction) or some time after the surgery (delayed reconstruction). Exactly when a woman decides to have reconstruction depends on her wishes and the specifics of her situation. She should discuss her options with her surgeon. Having a breast reconstructed can help a woman feel less self-conscious about how she looks and restore confidence in her sexuality.

Basically, there are two types of reconstruction. One uses artificial implants, and one uses skin and tissue from the woman's own body. The present day consensus is to perform immediate reconstruction with tissues from the woman's own body. In the modern era, every patient undergoing mastectomy should be offered the benefit of breast reconstruction.

Radiation Therapy

Like surgery, radiation therapy (also known as radiotherapy) is a local treatment for breast cancer. Using targeted, high-energy X-rays to stop cancer cells' ability to grow and divide, radiation therapy aims to get rid of cancer from the breast, chest, and axillary lymph nodes. The X-rays used during the procedure are similar to chest X-rays but are much higher in energy.

For women with early stage breast cancer, radiation therapy is most often performed following breast conserving surgery. Because undetectable microscopic cancer may be left in the breast after conserving surgery, radiation therapy is necessary to try to eliminate this disease and, therefore, reduce the chances of recurrence.

In addition to its role in breast conserving therapy, radiation therapy may also be used in certain cases on the axillary lymph nodes and on the chest wall following total mastectomy. Radiation therapy usually begins a few weeks after surgery after the wound has healed, though it is usually delayed if a patient is to receive chemotherapy. Most women who have had a total mastectomy do not need radiation therapy.

Adjuvant Systemic Treatment

While the goal of surgery and radiation therapy is to get rid of cancer "locally" in the breast, chest and armpit areas, the goal of systemic treatment in early stage breast cancer is to eliminate any cancer cells (called *micrometastases*) that may have spread from the breast tumor to other parts of the body as well as to eliminate any microscopic cancer cells that may remain in the local breast/lymph node area. Two types of systemic treatment are usually used for early stage breast cancer: **chemotherapy** and **hormone therapy**. These are called adjuvant (which means additional) therapies because they are used in addition to surgery and radiation and are given as part of the initial treatment plan. Adjuvant systemic therapy results in a decreased chance of the tumor coming back (recurrence) and also prolongs the life of the woman.

Except for some women with very small tumors (less than 1 cm) and with lymph nodes that do not have cancer, adjuvant therapy is almost always recommended for women with early-stage breast cancer. Which type of therapy a woman will get depends on many things, such as the woman's age, whether the tumor has estrogen receptors and the number of positive lymph nodes. Both chemotherapy and hormone therapy may be given alone, although many women receive both.

Chemotherapy uses drugs to kill cancer cells. It usually begins 3-4 weeks after the surgery and involves the use of a combination of drugs. The drugs are administered at three weekly intervals. This cycling allows the body a chance to rest and recover between treatments. It is usual to give six such cycles of chemotherapy. Chemotherapy is recommended in all pre-menopausal women. Post-menopausal women with estrogen receptor negative tumors also receive chemotherapy.

As most people are aware, chemotherapy has many side effects. Some are short-term side effects that develop during treatment and start to go away shortly after treatment is over. Others are long-term side effects that can persist for years. The frequency and severity of specific side effects can vary with the types of drugs used.

TABLE I

Some Short-Term Chemotherapy Side Effects

Nausea	Vomiting
Diarrhea	Hair loss (alopecia)
Mouth sores (stomatitis)	Low white blood cell count (neutropenia)
Low platelet count (thrombocytopenia)	Nerve pain (neuropathy)
Muscle pain (myalgia)	Temporary loss of period (amenorrhea)
Infection	Fatigue

The long-term side effects of chemotherapy range from the common to the very rare. Common long-term side effects of chemotherapy include early menopause and weight gain. Rare side effects include heart problems and leukemia

The most common **hormone therapy** for early stage breast cancer is the drug tamoxifen, although other therapies, such as suppression or removal of the ovaries, are sometimes used. Tamoxifen is usually prescribed for a period of five years for achieving maximal benefit. Tamoxifen has four established long-term side effects. It slightly increases the chance of developing endometrial cancer (cancer of the uterus), blood clots in the large veins (deep venous thrombosis), blood clots in the lungs (pulmonary emboli), and cataracts. While the prospect of such side effects can be frightening to some women, the risk of experiencing any one of them is very small and is far outweighed by the benefits of treating the cancer. Hormonal therapy is recommended for pre-menopausal and post-menopausal women with estrogen receptor positive tumors.

When the woman is to get both chemotherapy and hormonal therapy, usually chemotherapy precedes hormonal therapy.

Survival and Recurrence in Early Breast Cancer

Most women diagnosed with early stage breast cancer have a good outcome. Over 95 percent of women with stage I disease survive 5 years, and close to 90 percent survive 10 years those with stage II disease fare less well. Close to 85 percent survive 5 years, and approximately 65 percent survive 10 years. These numbers, however, are averages and do not apply directly to an individual woman.

Treatment of Locally Advanced Breast Cancer—Stage III

Recommended treatment for stage III cancers nearly always begins with chemotherapy rather than surgery. This chemotherapy (known as neoadjuvant, pre-operative, or primary chemotherapy) helps reduce the size of the tumors in the breast and lymph nodes so that surgery can more effectively remove them. Starting treatment with chemotherapy also has the advantage of being able to test which chemotherapy drugs will be most effective on a particular tumor. If the tumor does not get any smaller with one combination of drugs, other combinations can be tried.

The most common approach is to follow neoadjuvant

therapy with surgery—usually total mastectomy. If the tumor shrinks sufficiently, breast conserving surgery can be performed in selected cases. This is followed by an additional round of chemotherapy. Radiation therapy is then given as further local treatment. Women with estrogen receptor positive tumors then receive tamoxifen for a period of five years.

With chemotherapy, surgery and radiation, women with stage III breast cancer have a 50 to 60 percent chance of surviving five years after diagnosis. Women who respond to neoadjuvant chemotherapy to the extent of complete disappearance of the tumor do exceptionally well.

Treatment of Metastatic Breast Cancer—Stage IV

Most women who develop metastatic cancer do so after their initial treatment has failed, and cancer has returned. Only a small number of women (about 6-10 percent) have an initial diagnosis of metastatic disease.

As hard as it may be for women to hear, metastatic breast cancer cannot be cured. Unlike breast cancer that remains localized in the breast or lymph nodes, cancer that has spread to other organs cannot be completely eliminated. This does not mean, however, that it cannot be treated. With systemic and local therapy, some women with metastatic disease can live for many years, and ongoing research is constantly searching for new and better therapies for the disease.

The general approach to treating metastatic breast cancer focuses on maintaining a woman's quality of life while at the same time, lengthening her life. Balancing these two goals is the key to the treatment of metastatic breast cancer.

Treatment of Carcinoma In Situ (DCIS and LCIS)

Ductal Carcinoma In Situ (DCIS) is treated with either total mastectomy or breast conserving surgery plus radiation. Selected patients with favourable DCIS can be treated with conserving surgery alone. Because pure DCIS is contained within the ducts and does not have the potential to spread to the axillary nodes (as compared with invasive cancer), an axillary dissection is usually not performed as part of diagnosis and treatment. Women with DCIS should strongly consider taking tamoxifen for five years following their treatment.

LCIS raises the risk of cancer in both breasts, but because it is unlikely to turn into invasive cancer itself, its main management is observation. A woman with LCIS should see a caregiver regularly and be screened regularly for breast cancer. If invasive breast cancer develops, it can be diagnosed and treated early.

The Return of Breast Cancer (Recurrence)

The main goal of treatment for breast cancer is to keep the cancer from returning (recurrence). Because treatment is a very difficult and draining process, when it fails and the cancer returns, this can have a large emotional, as well as physical, effect on a woman. The tests and examinations done as part of regular follow-up help find cancer that has returned to the original area of surgery (local recurrence), as well as cancer that has spread to other parts of the body (distant recurrence). Regularly performing blood or other tests has not been shown to be an effective way to detect recurrence and is not a recommended part of follow-up care. Women who have been treated for breast cancer need to continue to see their doctors regularly. This follow-up care helps track the effectiveness of treatment and provides a time for women to share with their doctor any concerns they have about their breast cancer.

The goals of these regular visits are to help:

- Find any cancer that has returned to the breast, chest wall, or lymph nodes (local recurrence).
- Find breast cancer that has spread to other parts of the body (distant recurrence).
- Find in early stages any newly developed breast tumors.
- Find any side effects related to treatment (such as lymphedema or endometrial cancer).
- Provide continuing emotional and psychological support for the patient.

Recommended follow-up after breast cancer treatment includes both regular hospital visits and patient self-monitoring. At the hospital visits, a woman will have a physical examination, regular mammogram and pelvic examination; learn about symptoms she should be aware of; and be asked about any symptoms she's been having. Metastatic cancer is usually found because a woman develops symptoms (such as headaches, shortness of breath, bone pain and weight loss) and contacts her physician. Follow-up visits should also be used to share how a woman is coping emotionally and psychologically. In addition to discussing these issues with the surgeon, the patient can be referred to an appropriate support group or counselor, if she has not been referred already

Treating Breast Cancer in Pregnancy

There are special treatment considerations for pregnant women who have breast cancer, as certain therapies can have adverse effects on the fetus. Of all women under age 40 who have breast cancer, about 15 percent may be pregnant at the time of diagnosis. Cancer is often diagnosed at a more advanced stage in pregnant women than non-pregnant women, because the increased size and change in texture of the breast during pregnancy make smaller cancers difficult to detect. In addition, mammography is contraindicated in pregnant women. As a result, most cancers in pregnant women are first suspected during a clinical breast exam. Suspicious lumps can then be evaluated safely with ultrasound. Once diagnosed, total mastectomy is generally the recommended treatment for pregnant women who are in their first or second trimester and want to continue their pregnancy. Breast conserving surgery with radiation is usually not recommended, as radiation therapy can harm the fetus. Women in their third trimester can have breast conserving surgery and then put-off radiation therapy until after delivery. This will not affect their prognosis.

Chemotherapy is the only adjuvant therapy used during pregnancy, and even it cannot be administered without some risk to the fetus. The chances for chemotherapy-related birth defects are greatest in the first trimester. During the second and third trimesters, some chemotherapy drugs can be used. Women diagnosed in their third trimester usually put-off chemotherapy until after giving birth. Tamoxifen is not recommended at any point during pregnancy because of its risk to the fetus.

Prognosis for pregnant women with breast cancer is very similar to that of non-pregnant women, when stage of the cancer is taken into account. Although aborting a pregnancy can increase a woman's treatment options since the safety of the fetus is no longer a concern, it does not seem to affect prognosis.

APPENDIX I

Guidelines for Management of Chronic Obstructive Pulmonary Disease (COPD) in India, (PGI, Chandigarh)*

Introduction

Chronic Obstructive Pulmonary Disease (COPD) is a common problem encountered in medical practice. A review of studies available from India reveal the median prevalence of COPD is about 5% in men and 2.79% in women of over 30 years of age.

Definition

COPD, which includes two distinct pathophysiological processes as (chronic bronchitis and emphysema) is a condition characterized by airflow obstruction/limitation that is not fully reversible. It is associated with an abnormal inflammatory response of the lungs to noxious particles or gases especially tobacco smoke and air pollution—both indoor and outdoor. Chronic bronchitis manifests as chronic cough and sputum production for more than 3 months of a year for at least 2 consecutive years on most days. Emphysema presents with dyspnoea of insidious onset. The disease is gradually progressive leading to respiratory disability and death.

---

* These guidelines were developed to help in the management of COPD, especially at the Primary Care Level with standard criteria for management and referral strategies. These Guidelines were developed under the WHO-GOI Biennium (2002-2003) at the consensus Workshop organized by the Department of Pulmonary Medicine, Postgraduate Institute of Medical Education & Research, Chandigarh, in December 2002. The Workshop was attended by experts/consultants from National Institutes, Medical Colleges, and representatives from Government and private health services. The Indian Council of Medical Research, Indian Chest Society, National College of Chest Physicians, and the American College of Chest Physicians were also involved in the preparation of these guidelines.

Risk Factors

1. Tobacco smoking—most important
2. Exposure to environmental tobacco smoke (passive smoking).
3. Use of solid fuel (dried dung, wood, etc.) for combustion.
4. Outdoor air pollution (vehicular, industrial & occupational exhausts, dusts and fumes).

Symptoms

1. Chronic cough with sputum production; present on most days for at least 3 months/year for 2 or more consecutive years; cough is rarely nocturnal.
2. Dyspnoea persistent and progressive, worsening on exertion.

Physical Examination

A. *Findings Supportive of COPD*

1. Features of hyperinflation: barrel shaped chest, increased antero-posterior diameter, low placed diaphragm, i.e. downward displaced upper border of liver dullness and absence of cardiac dullness on percussion.
2. Diminished intensity of breath sounds with prolonged expiration.
3. Prolonged forced expiratory time; pursed lip breathing.

B. *Exclusion of Alternate Diagnoses Especially Asthma*

It is also important to exclude tuberculosis in all patients with sputum production. Look for:

1. Presence of localized physical findings.
2. Evidence of fibrocavitory disease/malignancy.

C. Complications of COPD

Look for evidence of (i) chronic cor pulmonale with or without right heart failure (raised jugular venous pressure, pedal oedema, loud P2), and (ii) respiratory failure (cyanosis, flaps, altered sensorium).

Investigations

1. Sputum for acid fast bacilli (AFB) (thrice): recommended for all patients presenting with chronic cough and expectoration.
2. Chest radiograph: as far as possible, should be obtained at primary care level to exclude and/or recognize alternate diagnoses and problems. It should always be done at the secondary care level.

Spirometry: if available, should be offered. Patients should also be referred for spirometry if the diagnosis is in doubt. Spirometry should be made available at least at the secondary care (district hospital) level.

Diagnosis

I. Provisional

The diagnosis of COPD should be considered in any patient with (1) history of exposure to risk factors (esp. tobacco smoking), and (2) suggestive symptoms.

II. Confirmatory

Spirometry is essential for confirmation of diagnosis of COPD. The presence of a post-bronchodilator forced expiratory volume1 $(FEV)_1$ < 80% of the predicted value in combination with an FEV_1/FVC < 70% confirms the presence of airflow limitation that is not fully reversible. Where necessary, reversibility of airflow obstruction should be excluded (defined as > 200 ml and 12% increase in FEV_1 or FVC (forced vital capacity) after bronchodilator). FEy1 value should be used for grading of severity of COPD. Other diseases, especially tuberculosis should be excluded. *If sputum is positive for (AFB), patient should be referred to the nearest*

Centre under Revised National Tuberculosis Control Programme. If no Centre is available, anti-tubercular treatment should be started as per standard guidelines.

Management

A. Assess the disease severity and start treatment depending upon the stage. Refer to Tables 1 and 2 for details.

TABLE I

Staging and Management Principles

	0 - At risk	*I - Mild*	*II - Moderate*	*III - Severe*
Risk Factors	Tobacco Smokers			
Symptoms[a]	No dyspnoea Mucoid expectoration	Dyspnoea on unaccustomed activity or climbing two flights of stairs	Dyspnoea on accustomed activity	Dyspnoea at rest
Signs		Nil or minimal	Chest hyperinflation Use of accessory muscles (mild) Wheezing	Moderate to severe use of necessary muscles Near absence of breath sounds Respiratory failure Evidence of right heart failure
Six minute walk test[b]		> 200 m	100-200 m	< 100 m
Peak expiratory flow (PEF)	Normal	50-70%	30-50%	< 30%
Spiromeery[c]	Normal	FEV_1/FVC < 70% FEV_1 > 80% predicted	FEV_1/FVC < 70% FEV_1 < 30-80% predicted	FEV_1/FVC < 70% FEV_1 < 30% predicted
Treatment[d]	Tobacco cessation	Short acting bronchodilators, when needed	Regular treatment with one/more bronchodilators (Table 2) Pulmonary rehabilitation	As in II, plus Inhaled corticosteroids[e] Treatment of complications

a Cough and expectoration are present at all stages.
b Performed by measuring distance covered in 6 minutes when patient walks at his/her own speed (under physician supervision).
c Important for good staging and definitive diagnosis. PEP (peak expiratory flow) is a good and cheap substitute for spirometry.
d Smoking cessation, patient education and other components of respiratory rehabilitation at all stages.
e Add if significant response of symptoms and lung function to a six week trial, or if repeated exacerbations. Inhaled corticosteroids are administered in a daily dose of 400-800 ug (or even more) of Beclomethasone propionate or equivalent.

TABLE 2

Commonly used Bronchodilator Drugs in India

Drugs	*Metered dose/ dry powder inhalers (μg)*	*Oral*
Beta agonists		
Saibutamol	100 200 SOS/tid/qid	2 4 mg tid/qid
Terbutaline	250 500 SOS/tid/qid	2.5 5 mg tid
Salmeterol	2550 bid	—
Formoterol	6 12 bid	—
Bambuterol	—	10 20 mg/day
Anticholinergics		
Ipratropium	40 50 rid/qid	—
Tiotropium	18 36 od	—
Methylxanthines		
Aminophylline	—	225 450 mg/day
Theophyllins	—	200 600 mg/day

B. Assess the risk factors and other complications. Advise and help to quit smoking. Smoking cessation is the most important and effective step. Standard guidelines for this purpose are summarized in Table 3.

C. Manage Acute Exacerbation if any

(i) Increase the dose and/or frequency of the existing bronchodilator therapy. Add new bronchodilators, drugs that are not being taken by the patient.

FIG. 1

Algorithm for Diagnosis and Management of COPD at Different Levels of Health Care

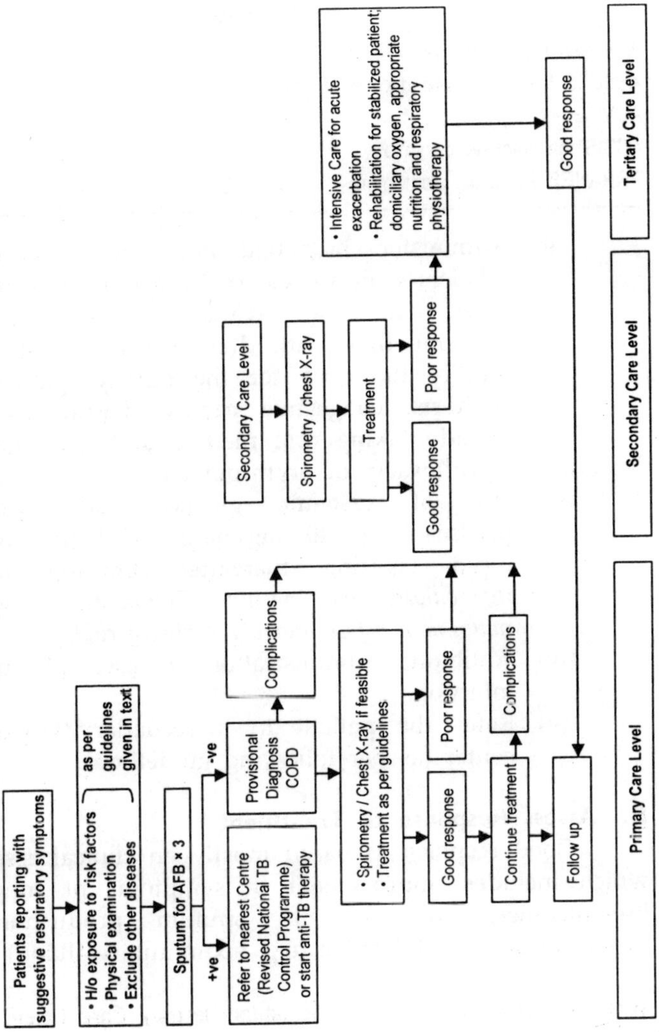

TABLE 3

Guidelines for Doctors on Smoking Cessation Follow the 5A Strategy

ASK about tobacco use
ASSESS the status and degree of use
ADVISE to stop
ASSIST in smoking cessation
ARRANGE follow-up programme

(ii) Administer bronchodilators by metered dose inhalers with spacers or by nebulization in severe cases. If not available, use intravenous aminophylline with due attention to its toxicity modify the dose for the elderly, patients with cirrhosis, congestive cardiac failure and those already taking oral methyl-xanthines, cimetidine, ciprofloxacin or erythromycin.

(iii) Use of systemic glucocorticoids, e.g. oral prednisolone (40 mg/day) for 5-10 days with rapid tapering thereafter. *Carefully look for tuberculosis by sputum examination and chest radiograph before starting corticosteroids.*

(iv) Antibiotic administration in case of suspected infection.

(v) Refer the patient to a secondary/tertiary care center (as per following guidelines).

D. Assess Response to Treatment

Good response is based mostly on clinical assessment which includes improvement in symptoms of cough and breathlessness; reduction in sputum production, and increased exercise tolerance (e.g. six-minute walking).

When to refer the patient to Secondary/Tertiary Care Level?

1. Any patient with symptoms of cardiac or respiratory failure.
2. Those patients not responding to treatment at primary level.

3. The patients in whom alternate diagnoses are strongly suspected.
4. Patients requiring assistance in tobacco cessation and/or respiratory rehabilitation.

The patient should be referred to a center where diagnostic and other facilities, including spirometry and inpatient services, are available.

APPENDIX II

DISC SURGERY

DR. ANUPAM JINDAL*

ANATOMY OF THE LUMBAR SPINE

The Spinal Column and the Vertebrate

Your spinal column consists of 24 separate bones, called vertebrae, plus the five fused bones of the sacrum and four fused bones of the coccyx (often referred to as the "tail bone") (Fig. 1). The vertebrae are stacked one on top of another and can be divided into:

1. The *cervical* (neck) spine : the top seven vertebrae,
2. The *thoracic* (chest) spine : the middle 12 vertebrae, and
3. The *lumbar* (lower back) spine : the bottom five vertebrae.

Support for the Vertebral (Spine) Column

Attached to the vertebrae are muscles, tendons and a group of bands, called ligaments. Together, they support the spinal column and help to protect its delicate nerves.

The Role of the Vertebral (Spine) Column

Your spinal column enables you to walk upright. It is the central support for your upper body and carries the weight of your head, chest and arms. The vertebrae in the lumbar (or lower back) portion of your spine carry the

---

* M.Ch. (Neurosurgery), AIIMS, (Formerly Asstt. Prof. Neurosurgery, AIIMS), Consultant Neurosurgery. #787, FF, Sector 43A, Chandigarh.

majority of this weight. The constant pressure from this weight, even when you are simply sitting in a chair, is what usually leads to problems associated with the lower back.

The Role of the Intervertebral Discs

The bony vertebrae of your spinal column are separated from on another by "pads" of tough cartilage, called intervertebral discs (Fig. 2). These discs act like "Shock absorbers" during activity, allowing the spine to move freely. How a disc "ruptures" (bulges outward) is shown in the drawing to the right (Fig. 2) and will be discussed in detail on the following pages.

The Intervertebral Disc Nucleus

The centre of each intervertebral disc is made up of a gelatin-like substance (the nucleus), surrounded by a fibre-like outer lining (the annulus) (Fig. 3). As your body ages, the disc's nucleus begins to stiffen. This reduces flexibility and increases the chances that a disc may "rupture", especially in the lumbar spine which carries so much of your body's weight.

ANATOMY OF THE LUMBAR SPINE

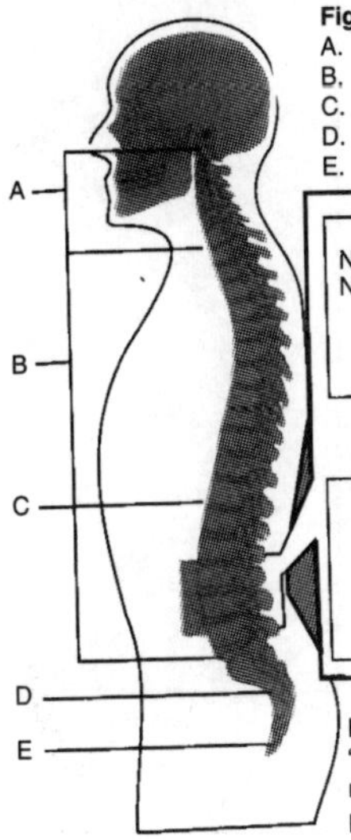

Figure 1 (left) : The spinal column is divided into the :
A. Cervical spine (7 vertebrae)
B. Thoracic spine (12 vertebrae)
C. Lumbar Spine (5 vertebrae)
D. Sacrum (5 fused bones)
E. Coccyx (4 fused bones)

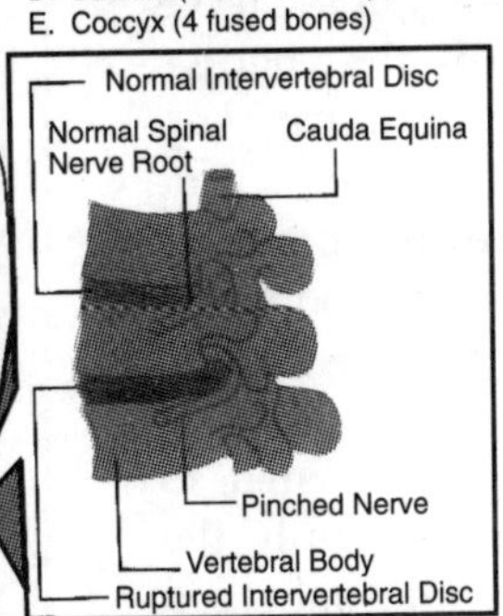

Figure 2 (above) : When an intervertebral disc "ruptures" (bulges outward), it can press a spinal nerve root(s) against the bony vertebra causing pain in your lower back and legs(s)

ANATOMY OF THE LUMBAR SPINE

The Spinal Canal

The *spinal cord*, which begins at the base of the brain and runs within the spinal canal, ends in the lumbar spine area in a bundle of nerves known as the cauda equina. The *spinal canal* runs through the centre of the spinal column and protects the spinal cord and other delicate spinal nerves.

Figures 3: View of a vertebra, the cauda equina, spinal nerve roots and the intervertebral disc.

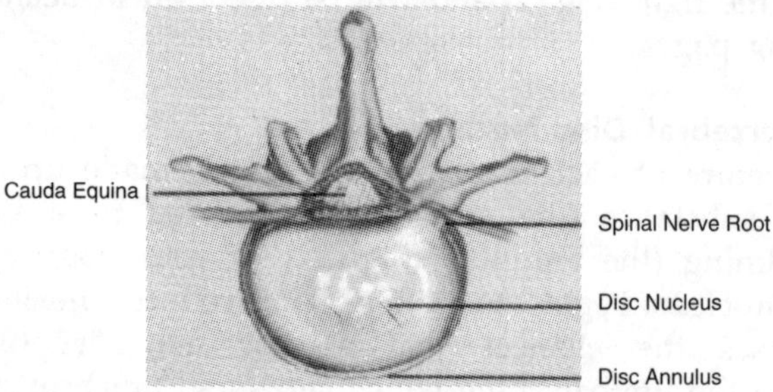

The Spinal Nerve Roots

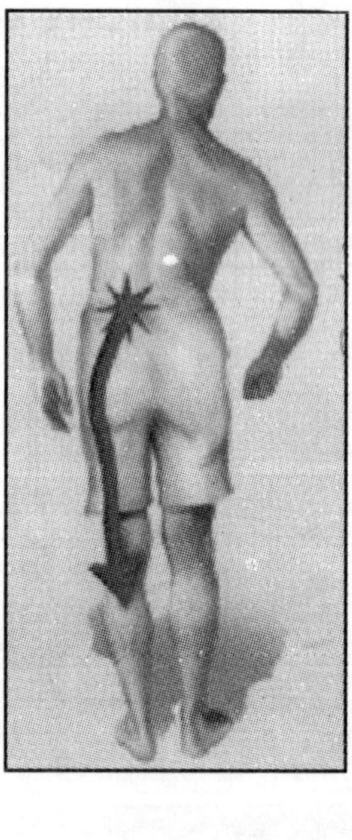

At each vertebral level, a pair of nerves branch off from the spinal cord or the cauda equina (one to the left and one to the right). These spinal nerve roots are part of the body's "electrical" system, carrying "current" (for sensation and movement) to specific parts of the body. The nerve roots are protected by an "insulated" covering in the same way a "live" electrical line is coated to prevent direct contact with the bare wire. A nerve root damaged by a ruptured disc may have all or part of its "insulation" rubbed off at the point of injury. Prior to surgery there is no way of telling how much has been rubbed-off or how much damage has been done to the nerve (the body's "live electrical wire").

WHEN A DISC RUPTURES

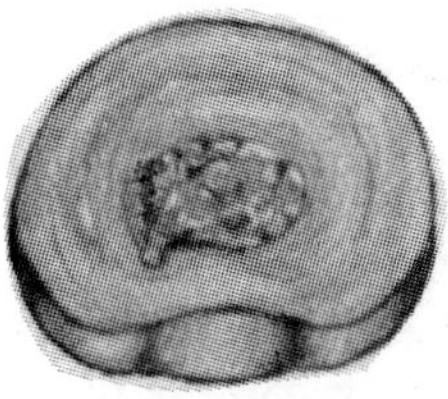

Disc protrusion

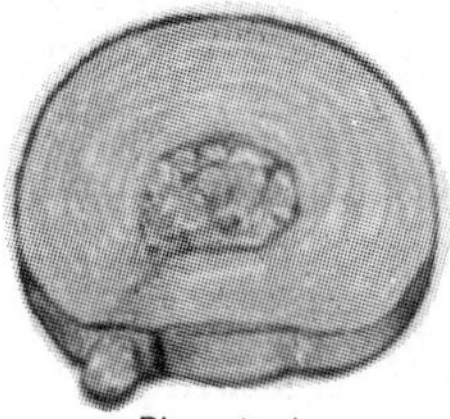

Disc extrusion

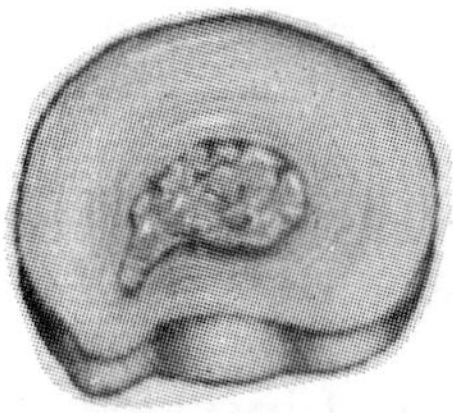

Disc herniation

What Happens When a Disc Ruptures?

When the outer lining (annulus) of a disc "tears", its cente (the nucleus) may rupture and press a spinal nerve(s) against the bony surface of a vertebra (Fig. 4). This condition is often referred to as a ruptured disc. You could think of it as having a tube of toothpaste with a crack in it. Exert pressure on the cracked tube (disc annulus) and toothpaste (disc nucleus) flows out the crack. Even pressure from everyday activities can push the disc's nucleus through the ruptured annulus and pinch a spinal nerve root(s).

What Causes a Disc to Rupture?

As we've discussed, your lumbar spine supports the weight of your entire upper body and it under stress every day. Simple "wear and tear" or the effects of aging can contribute to a disc rupture. In some cases, the rupture happens during the course of normal, everyday activities. In other cases, it occur as the result of a specific injury. Usually there is no way to "prevent" it from occurring, however, you can reduce your risk by staying in good physical condition and by using proper lifting techniques.

What are the Symptoms of a Ruptured Disc?

When a lumbar spinal nerve is pinched, you may experience pain in your lower back, pain or numbness in one or both of your feet. The pain can come from the pressure on the nerve, the swelling within the nerve (caused by the pressure) or injury to the nerve itself. Taking pain medication or drugs which reduce the swelling may provide relief, but healing may not occur as long as the nerve itself remains pinched. It's similar to having your finger caught in a door. An aspirin may help to ease the pain, but healing won't begin until the door is opened and your finger is no longer being pinched.

How is a Ruptured Lumbar Disc Diagnosed?

The diagnosis of a ruptured lumbar disc is based on:

1. Your history of back and/or leg pain.
2. A physical examination of your back and legs, and
3. Diagnostic tests, which may include spine X-rays, an MRI scan, a CAT scan or a myelogram. (Each of these examinations has a specific purpose).

YOUR TREATMENT OPTIONS . . .

Treatment Options

There are a number of treatment options for a reptured lumbar disc, each **accompanied** by its own set of risks and benefits.

The four basic approaches are:

1. Taking Time

For some patients, all that is required in order to heal and recover is time.

2. Taking Medication

For others, medication may reduce the inflammation or

ease the pain in the affected area and thereby provide relief from their symptoms.

3. Using Physical Therapy

For some, physical measures such as physical therapy (or gentle exercise) may provide relief and aid in the recovery from a reptured disc.

4. Having Surgery

For those patients whose reptured disc is causing a "pinched" nerve, a MED procedure often is the recommended treatment.

When a MED Procedure is not an Option

The severity of your symptoms (pain, weakness, lack of mobility) and your general health and physical condition will play an important part in determining when surgery is not an option for you. In general, surgery is not an option when:

1. Your back and leg pain is not caused by a ruptured disc.
2. There is a medical reason which prevents you from having surgery.
3. Medication which reduces swelling or relieves pain would provide you with adequate relief.
4. Physical measures would improve your condition.

When a MED Procedure is an Option

Lumbar micro-endoscopic dissectomy (MED) is usually recommended only when specific conditions are met. In general, surgery is recommended when a reptured disc is pinching a spinal nerve root(s) and you have:

1. Leg pain which limits your normal daily activities.
2. Weakness in your leg(s) or feet.
3. Numbness in your extremities.
4. Impaired bowel and/or bladder function.

The Risks of having Surgery

Some of the more common risks of having any surgery

include excessive bleeding, infection or a negative reaction to anesthesia. Certain unforeseen circumstances could even lead to death. Clinical experience and scientific calculation indicate that these risks are low, but surgery is still a human effort. You should feel free to ask any question you have about your specific risk factors.

Since the MED procedure involves surgery in and around the spine, further nerve damage is a possibility. In some cases the nerve is already so damaged that the surgical procedure required to simply each the nerve could be the "straw that breaks the camel's back." The end result could be numbness, paralysis or a loss of bowel and bladder control. (However, deciding not to have surgery may have exactly the same consequences). Your decision should be based on a weighing of the risks of having surgery *versus* the risks of not having surgery.

The Benefits of having Surgery

You can think of surgery as the first step in the healing and recovery process. It can help relieve your pain. It also may help you begin the process of regaining some of the lost mobility in your extremities.

... AND THEIR RISKS AND BENEFITS

The MED Procedure and its Specific Benefits

The MED procedure is an operation on the lumbar spine performed using a surgical endoscope and microsurgical techniques. The MED procedure requires only a very small incision and will remove only that portion of your ruptured disc which is "pinching" one or more spinal nerve roots. The recovery times for this particular surgery is usually much less than is required for traditional lumbar surgery.

Your Chances for Success

Your level of healing will be determined by your age, your general health and the severity of the damage to your spinal nerve, as well as your attitude and your willingness to work at recovery.

TABLE OF CONTENTS

Making Your Decision

When you consider your options, keep in mind the impact your condition has on your way of life and carefully weigh the risks and benefits of having surgery against the risks and benefits of not having surgery.

The decision of yours!

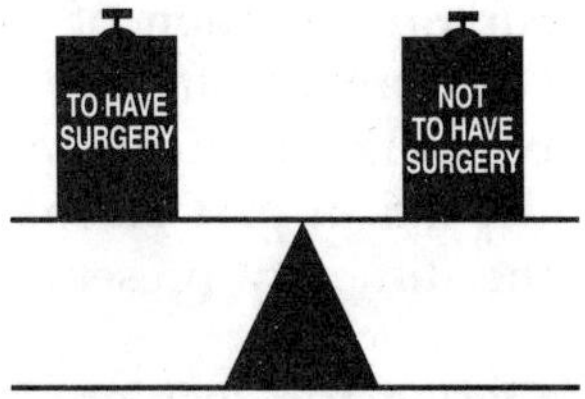

THE SURGICAL PROCEDURE

The Surgeon's Role

Your surgeon will (1) review your neurological history and examination, (2) Review your diagnostic studies (such as a myelogram, CAT scan or MRI, (3) Plan a surgical approach, and (4) review the procedure with you.

Your Role

You must have a thorough understanding of the diagnosis (what is causing your back and/or leg symptoms) and the risks and benefits of the proposed surgery. Once you are confident that surgery is the correct option for you, turn your thoughts to the future and the recovery process.

The Operation

In the operating room a K-wire is passed under floroscopy control at the level of offending disc. Then a series of dilators is passed over this K-wire and then a working channel is passed over these dilators. Through this opening, your surgeon will insert the endoscope and surgical instruments. Because the work is viewed through an endoscope, this approach requires a relatively small incision. Guided by diagnostic studies, your surgeon may remove a small portion of bony material from the back of your vertebra. Once this material is removed, the surgeon can locate the exact area where the nerve root is being pinched.

Identifying the Cause of the Pressure

Once the "pinched" nerve is located, the extent of the pressure on the nerve can be determined. Using endoscopic microsurgical procedures, your surgeon will remove the ruptured portion of the disc and any disc fragments which have broken-off from the main disc (Fig. below). The amount of work required to complete your MED procedure will depend in part on the number of disc fragments present and the difficulty presentation in finding and removing them.

Closing the Incision

The operation is completed when the endoscope is removed and the incision is closed with suture materials and a bandage.

The Healing and Recovery Process

Once the ruptured disc has been removed, healing can begin. Healing is body's natural process can begin. Healing is body's natural process of restoring its damaged tissues to a normal, or nearly normal condition. Healing occurs on its own, but is influenced by such factors as general good health, physical fitness, nutrition and rest. Recovery is the process during which you work at becoming well. You must commit yourself to staying in good health (exercising), maintaining a positive mental attitude and following your physician's instructions.

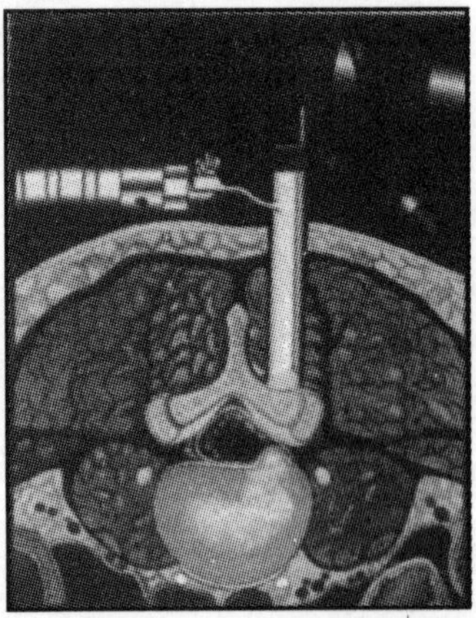

The Surgeon uses microscopic instruments to remove the portion of the ruptured disc which is pinching the cauda equina or the spinal nerve oot.

WHAT TO EXPECT AFTER SURGERY

Have Realistic Expectations

Recognize that healing and recovery will not happen overnight. It is a process. You may find that much of your progress will be like taking "two steps forward and one step back." Accept it! And then do all that you can to make sure your steps "forward" are large ones and your steps "backward" are small ones.

Be Patient and Persistent

During the recovery period in the hospital and at home, try to rebuild your strength gradually. Rest when you feel fatigued—but be persistent in your efforts.

It is important for you to recognize that we all heal at a different rate. The *speed at which you will recover depends in part on your age, your general level of health, your overall physical fitness and your mental attitude*. Generally you will heal more slowly if you are over weight, out of shape or smoke, or if you are diabetic or have other pre-existing medical problems.

Expect some Pain after Surgery

It is normal to have some pain after any operation. After a MED procedure, there may be some leg "aching" which occurs as the nerve(s) attempts to heal. You may feel some muscle spasms across your back and down your leg(s). And if there was inflammation in the nerve root, some pain persist until this inflammation diminishes. You will be given appropriate medication to control your pain, relieve back spasms and reduce inflammation.

Be Prepared for Some Emotional Changes

It is not unusual to feel tired and discouraged for several days following surgery. These feelings may be your body's natural reaction to the cutback of extra hormones it generated during surgery. Although some emotional letdown can be expected, you must not let it get in the way of your recovery. Don't look back at past problems. It is important for you to look at even the smallest positive steps you make as progress towards your recover goal.

Develop a Positive Mental Attitude

You should begin to work on a positive mental attitude even *before* the surgery is performed. Direct your energies toward the solution of your problem, rather than worrying about what caused your problem. Don't be discouraged by minor setbacks during the recovery process. *Concentrate on the progress you make, and will continue to make in the future.*

Commit to a Healthy Lifestyle

Now is the time to commit yourself to a healthier lifestyle. You can begin by taking these important steps:

Watch your weight: If you are overweight, You must gradually return to your proper weight. Crash diets rarely work. Commit yourself to better eating habits and stay with them for the rest of your life.

Become more active: Your physician will tell you when you can resume normal physical activities after surgery. Make up your mind now that you will develop a regular aerobic exercises routine, such as walking, swimming or riding a bike. However, always check with your physician before starting any exercise program.

Going Home from the Hospital

In general, hospital stays are becoming shorter, especially for endoscopic procedures. Even though you may feel somewhat uncomfortable at the time you are released, your physician usually will allow you to go home when:

1. Your vital signs are stable.
2. You can walk on your own.
3. You can eat without having nausea.
4. You have resumed normal bladder activity.
5. Your wound is healing.

Recovering at Home

Since you are at home and you begin to resume your normal activities, follow the guidelines listed below (and contact your physician's office if you have any question):

Exercise: Try to do as much as you can. Daily walking is the best exercise. Set reasonable goals, but gradually increase the distance you walk each day. *Check with your physician before starting any exercise program.*

Sitting and standing: Do not sit or stand for long periods of time. If you have muscle spasms in your back or pain in your leg(s), changing positions frequently should help.

Sleeping: Rest when you feel fatigued, but do not spend all of your time in bed. Please note that waking up with a "stiff' back is not uncommon. For relief, try taking a short walk or a warm shower. If you do not have a firm mattress, invest in one-it is important for proper back support.

Caring for your Incision: Wash your incision gently and pat it dry. If you see any increased redness, swelling or drainage, notify your physician.

Medication

You should gradually reduce the amount of pain medication you take. Begin by increasing the amount of time between pills, and then reduce the number of pills taken each time. A certain amount of discomfort can be expected until the swelling goes down and the nerve sensitivity decreases. Substitute moist heat, gentle exercise and short rest periods for pain medication whenever possible.

Preventive Measures

The best way to avoid the recurrence of a reptured disc is to maintain a healthy lifestyle. It is important that you:

1. Eat a *well-balanced diet* in order to aid proper healing (avoid foods high in calories and fat content).
2. Continue to eat a healthy diet in the future to reach and maintain your proper body weight.
3. Get the *proper amount of sleep.*
4. Participate in some form of *regular aerobic exercise* (such as walking, swimming, riding a bike, etc.).
5. Take *extra care when lifting, bending or twisting.*
6. Take *care of other health problems.* (Such as heart disease, etc.).

APPENDIX III

NASAL ALLERGIES

—CIPLA

Nasal Allergy is also called Allergic Rhinitis. It is the most common allergy encountered in clinical practice and constitutes more than 50% of all allergies seen in India. One person in every six suffers from the disease, making it the most prevalent among all chronic diseases and its incidence is steadily increasing. Allergic rhinitis has a sizeable economic impact associated with healthcare utilization and patient's reduced productivity. Nasal symptoms are often demeaned; however, their prevalence and effect on quality of life, justify an aggressive but rational approach. It must also be acknowledged that rhinitis and asthma frequently co-exist, with rhinitis appearing first in about 45% of the patients. Besides, it is well documented that adequate nasal treatment can improve pulmonary functions.

Allergic Rhinitis and its Effect on Quality of Life (QOL)

The indirect costs associated with allergic rhinitis are

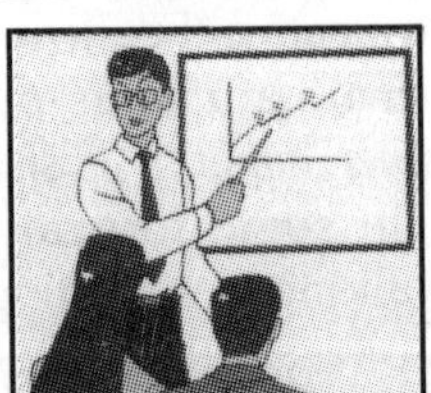

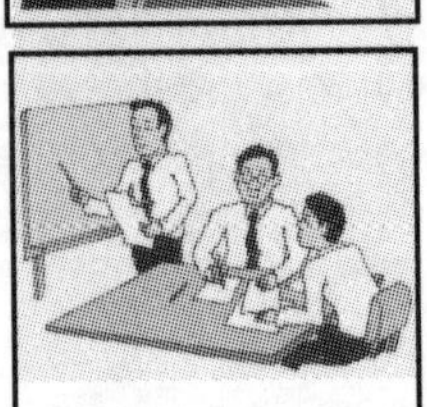

linked to factors such as QOL, work productivity, learning, cognitive functioning, decision-making, and self-perception. All these factors must be evaluated as they are important components that affect patient's lives, socialization (such as learning or interaction with others), economics (e.g., work productivity, decision-making), and their general sense of well-being.

Allergic Rhinitis and its Impact in the Classroom and Workplace

Classroom productivity or cognitive (mental) ability can be evaluated with several different parameters reflecting a person's ability to learn, recall or process information. The Work Productivity and Activity Impairment Questionnaire results showed moderate-to-severe impairment in classroom productivity, and ability to do daily activities. This impairment was significant enough for nearly 25% of the patients missed time from work or school.

Allergic Rhinitis and Self-perception

Young people with allergic rhinitis especially have a general feeling of malaise and feel limited in their ability to perform daily activities. In a study of 5,938 students 15 to 19 years of age, 1,458 (24%) claimed to have had Allergic Rhinitis/Allergic Conjunctivitis in the past, with pollen being the most common allergen cited. Students selected statements in a questionnaire reflecting their attitudes regarding their symptoms. Students with allergic rhinitis registered a high agreement with the descriptives of "feeling tired" and "unattractive" because of allergic rhinitis.

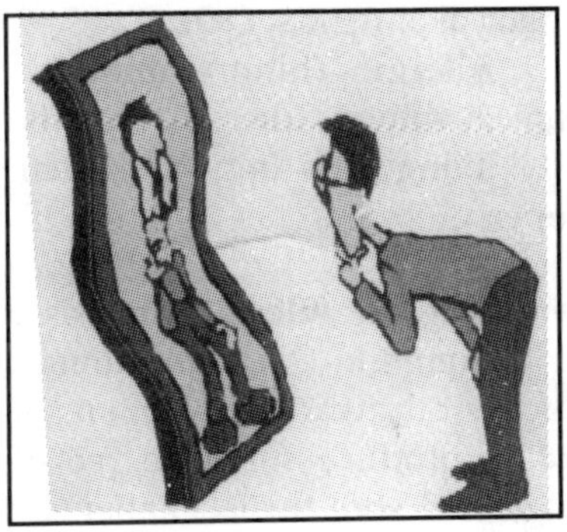

The Mechanisms underlying Allergic Rhinitis

A topic diseases like allergic rhinitis and asthma are generally caused by a sustained overproduction of Immunoglobulin E (IgE) in response to common environmental antigens such as pollen, moulds, house dust mite, animal dander and fungal spores. Basically, the IgE that is specific to the causative allergen binds to the IgE receptor on the surface of the mast cell and upon re-exposure to allergen cross linking of the IgE by allergen results in the release of a range of mediators like histamine, leukotrienes and prostaglandins leading to manifestation of the immediate hypersensitivity type responses.

Allergic rhinitis is characterized by typical symptoms of rhinorrhoea, sneezing, itching and nasal blockage, usually starting in early childhood with the symptoms peaking in the second, third and fourth decades of life. However, an onset of this disease in infancy or later in adults is not quite uncommon. A genetic background, an abnormal T cell response, and environmental pollution are among the strongly suggested determinants.

Although this condition is not life-threatening, it can significantly interfere with daily activities and negatively impact a patient's QOL.

Allergic rhinitis mimics the common cold in many respects. Since, allergic rhinitis influences many aspects of daily living it is important that it be diagnosed and treated properly.

Identifying an Allergic Rhinitis Patient

Common cold symptoms vary somewhat depending on which viral invader is responsible. However, virtually all cold viruses produce some degree of nasal blockage, runny nose, cough and sore throat. Patients may also experience headache or other bodyaches, occasional sneezing, weakness, dizziness, and postnasal drip. One or more family members, co-workers or playmates of the patient may also have the condition. Symptoms may occur 3-4 times yearly, each lasting for a period of 2-3 days (sneezing, sore throat) to as long as 2 weeks (cough, nasal discharge, postnasal drip, throat clearing).

Differentiating Allergic Rhinitis from the Common Cold

The Common Cold	*Allergic Rhinitis*
Gradual onset; slow progression	Sudden onset
—	Nasal pruritus & Itch
Sneezing is infrequent & deep in an attempt to clear bronchial or nasal congestion	Bouts of sneezing on allergen exposure; relatively quiet
—	Can cause ophthalmic problems
—	Watery discharge & tearing
Not likely to cause hyposmia and anosmia	More likely to cause hyposmia and anosmia

Similarities between Allergic Rhinitis and the Common Cold

Allergic Rhinitis	Rhinorrhoea	Nasal Congestion	Sneezing
The Common Cold	Rhinorrhoea	Nasal Congestion	Sneezing

Complications of Allergic Rhinitis

The common cold is a self-limiting condition for most patients, although some develop complications, such as otitis media and sinus infection. Allergic rhinitis is more likely to produce complications because of its recurrence. Patients who have perennial allergic rhinitis may be affected virtually constantly. Thus, allergic rhinitis is now recognized as a risk factor for the development of conditions such as asthma, sinusitis, otitis media and nasal polyps.

Interrelationship of Allergic Rhinitis and Associated Airway Disease

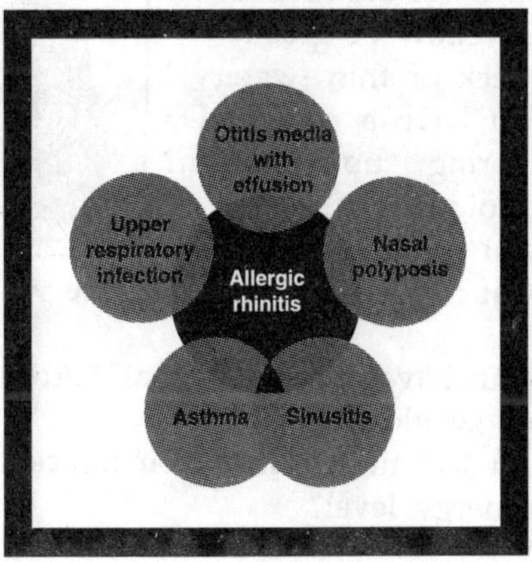

Pattern of Symptoms for Allergic Rhinitis vs. other Upper Respiratory Disorders

Symptom	*Allergic Rhinitis*	*Flu*	*Sinusitis*
Sneezing	+	+	
Rhinorrhoea	+ Clear	+	+ Purulent
Nasal Congestion	+/	+	+
Postnasal Drip	+	+	
Impaired Taste/Smell	+/-	+/-	+
Conjunctivitis	+/-		
Pruritus of Eyes, Ears, Nose or Throat	+		
Headaches		+	+/- Frontal sinuses
Fever		+ High-grade	+
Non-productive Cough		+	+/-
Productive Cough			
Sore throat		+	

Probe the Patient to Obtain Information about the Specific Symptoms

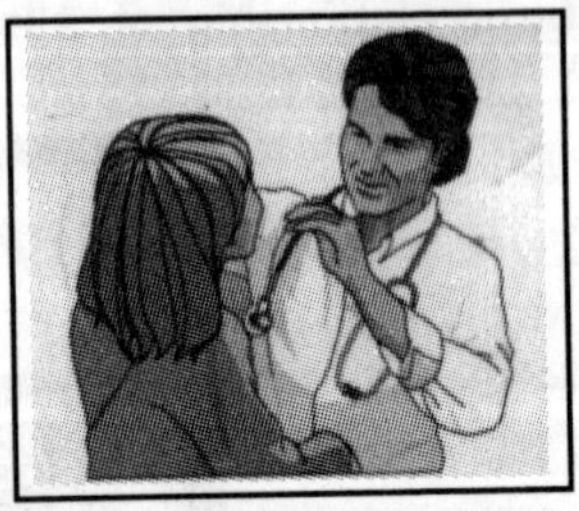

- Describe your symptoms.
- Is your nasal drainage clear, white, yellow or green?
- Is it thick or thin (watery)?
- Do you have a cough? Do you bring up sputum? What colour is it?
- Are you running a fever? If so, what is your temperature? Are you having any chills?
- Do you have a sore throat? Are you having trouble swallowing?
- Do you feel tired? Have you noticed a change in your energy level?

- Are you experiencing any muscle aches and pain?

Assess the Pattern of Symptoms

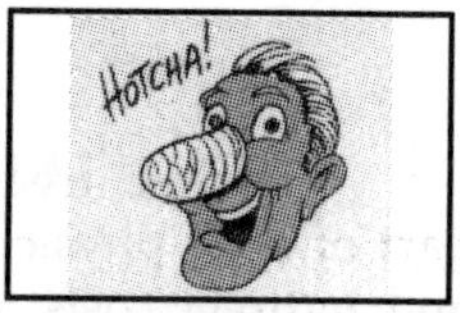

- How often do these symptoms occur?
- Do you notice a change in your symptoms when you are in different places, such as home, work or school?
- Do you notice a difference in your symptoms when you stay inside all day long or when you work or play outside? Are your symptoms worse during certain times of the day?
- Do you notice a change in your symptoms when you conduct specific activities, such as cooking, cleaning, gardening, etc?

Screen for Environmental Triggers

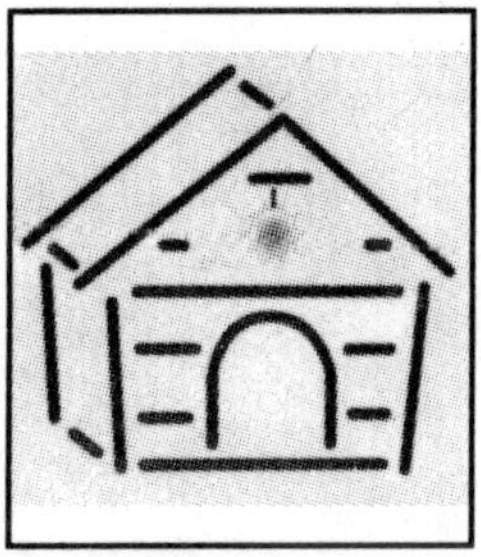

- hat type of flooring do you have in your home?
- How is your home heated and cooled? Do you open your windows?
- Do you have a ceiling fan in your bedroom?
- Do you have a pet? Does it stay indoors or outdoors?
- Does it sleep in your bedroom? Who grooms the pet?

Assess Medication Use

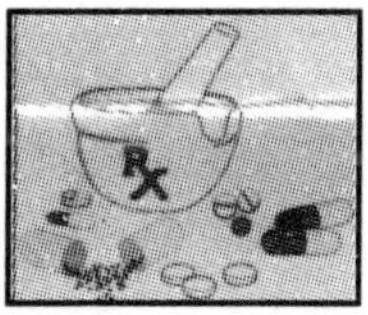

- Do you take medications regularly for these symptoms? If so:
- When was the last time medications were required?

- Did these medications help alleviate your symptoms?
- Did you experience any adverse effects with these medications?
- Show me how you use your nasal inhaler?

CONCLUSION

Effective treatment and greater understanding on the part of both physicians and patients can help to reduce direct and indirect costs as well as to lessen the impact of allergic rhinitis on QOL for both patients and society. Since, allergic rhinitis influences many aspects of daily living it is important that it be diagnosed and treated properly.

APENDIX IV

ORAL HEALTH

The important contribution of oral health to general community health and well-being has been highlighted in resolutions adopted at the World Health Assembly (WHA) and Regional Committees. However, the impact of these resolutions had been limited.

Previous approaches to oral health in Africa have failed to recognize the epidemiological priorities of the Region or to identify reliable and appropriate strategies to address them. Efforts have consisted of the provision of unplanned, *ad hoc* and spasmodic curative oral health services, which in most cases are poorly distributed and only reach affluent or urban communities.

Oral health systems are also characterized by the predominance of dentists, most of whom are in private practice in urban settings. Where public or private oral health services do function, they are treatment-oriented, mainly providing for the relieve of pain and sepsis and occasionally other curative forms of care. In September 1998, the WHO Regional Committee for Africa a disproportionate amount of oral disease which has grave and often fatal consequences. Some of these diseases seem to be growing in region there is prevalence as a result of the massive social disruption on the continent. Although many oral diseases oral health describes the well-being of the oral cavity, including the dentition and its supporting structures and tissues. It is the absence of disease and the optimal functioning of the mouth and its tissues, in a manner which helps to preserve high levels of self-esteem. Oral diseases affect all human beings irrespective of location, country, nationality, race or colour. In the African are not always life-threatening, they too are important public health problems because of their high prevalence, public demand and their impact on individuals and society in terms of pain, discomfort, social and functional limitations and handicap, and the effect on the quality of life. In addition, the financial impact on the individual and community is very high adopted a ten year (1999-2008) oral health strategy for the African Region [document (AFR/RC48/9) as well as a resolution (AFRO/RC48/R5)]. This strategy provides technical and managerial orientations that countries can use to streamline oral health services to efficiently and effectively deliver interventions that are affordable and that match the oral health needs of the community. It represents a new approach that has the potential to fundamentally improve community oral health in the African Region.

The Importance of Brushing

The single best way to remove harmful plaque—a thin, sticky film of bacteria—from teeth and gums is to brush teeth regularly and properly.

What is the Proper Technique for Teeth Brushing?

Because every mouth is different, there is more than one technique of brushing that has proven to be effective. Deciding which technique is most appropriate for you depends largely on your teeth position and gum condition. Consult your physician and/or dentist to determine which brushing technique is most appropriate for your mouth.

Generally, most dentists recommend a circular technique for brushing. This includes brushing only a small group of teeth at a time—gradually covering the entire mouth. The importance of maintaining a circular or elliptical motion is emphasized as using a back and forth motion may cause the following:

- a receded gum surface,
- an exposed and tender root surface, and
- a wearing down of the gum line.

Instead, dentists recommend the following method:

Step 1

Place the toothbrush beside your teeth at a 45-degree angle.

Step 2

Gently brush teeth only a small group of teeth at a time (in a circular or elliptical motion) until the entire mouth is covered.

Step 3

Brush the outside of the teeth, inside of the teeth, the chewing surfaces, and in between each tooth.

Step 4

Gently brush the tongue to remove bacteria and freshen breath.

Step 5

Repeat steps 1 through 4 at least twice daily, especially after meals and snacks.

What Type of Toothbrush should be Used?

A toothbrush head should be small—about 1 inch by 1/2 inch—and should have a handle suitable for firm grasping. The bristles of the brush should be soft, nylon, and rounded at the ends. This helps ensure that the brush bristles are reaching the spaces between the teeth as well as the surface. Some brushes are too abrasive and can wear down the enamel on teeth. Thus, in most cases, medium and hard bristles are not recommended.

How often is Brushing Necessary?

Generally, brushing is recommended twice a day for at least three to four minutes each time. Patients generally think they are brushing long enough, when, in fact, most people spend less than one minute brushing. In addition, it is generally better to brush 3 to 4 minutes twice a day instead of brushing quickly five or more times throughout the day.

Dentists advise brushing your teeth during the day while at work, school, or play. Keeping a toothbrush handy—

in your desk or backpack—increases the chances that you will brush during the day.

What is Toothpaste?

Also called dentifrice, toothpaste is comprised of the following cleaning ingredients (stated in approximate percentages):

- humectant and water—75 percent,
- abrasive—20 percent,
- foaming and flavoring agents—2 percent,
- pH buffers—2 percent,
- colouring agents, binders, and opacifiers Fluoride, is the most crucial ingredient in toothpaste. As long as the to—1.5 percent, and
- fluoride—24 percent.

Facts about Toothpaste

Brushing with toothpaste (particularly toothpaste with fluoride) helps to accomplish the following:

- remove plaque,
- resist decay,
- promote remineralization,
- clean and polish teeth,
- remove teeth stains, and
- freshen breath

Which Type of Toothpaste is Best?

Toothpaste contains fluoride, the brand, nor type (paste, gel, or powder) generally does not matter. All fluoride toothpastes work effectively to fight plaque and cavities, and clean and polish tooth enamel. The brand you choose should bear the ADA (American Dental Association) seal of approval on the container, which means that adequate evidence of safety and efficacy have been demonstrated in controlled, clinical trials. Some toothpastes offer tartar control pyrophosphates to prevent the build-up of soft calculus deposits on teeth, while others offer whitening formulas to safely remove stains making teeth brighter and shinier. But, contrary to clever advertising and popular belief, fluoride is the true active ingredient that works the hardest to protect your teeth.

What is Fluoride?

The fluoride ion comes from the element fluorine. Fluoride, either applied topically to erupted teeth, or ingested orally (called systemic fluoride) during tooth development, helps to prevent tooth decay, strengthen tooth enamel, and reduce the harmful effects of plaque. Fluoride also makes the entire tooth structure more resistant to decay and promotes remineralization, which aids in repairing early decay before the damage is even visible.

Where is Fluoride Found?

(FDA) classifies mouth rinses as either cosmetic or therapeutic, or a combination of the facts about mouth rinse.

Although mouth rinses may leave your breath feeling fresh, some mouth rinse formulas may actually be doing your mouth more harm than good. Mouth rinses do provide a fresh, crisp feeling after use, and many help to prevent cavities and plaque build-up, but, for some people, mouth rinses can be harmful. They may actually be masking the symptoms of an oral health disease or condition. With some conditions. such as periodontal disease, bad breath and a unpleasant taste in your mouth are the first (and sometimes only) indicators that something is wrong.

What are the Different Types of Mouthwash?

The US Food and Drug Administration too help remove oral debris before or after brushing:

- temporarily suppress bad breath,
- diminish bacteria in the mouth,
- refresh the mouth with a pleasant taste,
- it is important to note that most dentists are skeptical about the value of these antiplaque, mouth-rinsing products. Several studies have been conducted demonstrating the products' minimal effectiveness against reducing plaque. These

products should be used with caution, under the direction of an oral health care may be sold as prescription or over-the-counter,

- ❑ help remove oral debris before or after brushing,
- ❑ temporarily suppress bad breath,
- ❑ diminish bacteria in the mouth,
- ❑ refresh the mouth with a pleasant taste, and
- ❑ contain an added active ingredient that helps protect against some oral diseases.

Rinses of any kind should not be considered as substitutes for regular dental examinations and proper home care.

Mouthwashes Containing Alcohol

The ingredients of mouth washes vary, but some contain high levels of alcohol—ranging from 18 to 26 percent. This may produce a burning sensation in the cheeks, teeth, and gums, or may cause intoxication if swallowed or used excessively. For children, even small doses of these over-the-counter rinses can potentially be lethal.

When should Dental Care Begin?

Most pediatric dentists will agree that regular dental care should begin by one year of age, with a dental check-up at least twice each consecutive year for most children. Some children may need more frequent evaluations and care. In accordance with this recommendation, the following dental checklist for infants and toddlers has been provided by the American Academy of Pediatric Dentistry:

- ❑ During this time, the first tooth should appear. Consult the pediatric dentist for an examination.
- ❑ Brush teeth after each feeding birth to 6 months of age.
- ❑ Clean the infant's mouth with gauze after feedings and at bedtime.
- ❑ Consult your child's pediatrician regarding fluoride supplements.
- ❑ Regulate feeding habits (bottle feeding and breastfeeding).

Six to 12 Months of Age

- ❑ And at bedtime with a small, soft-bristled brush.
- ❑ As the child begins to walk, stay alert of potential dental and/or facial injuries.
- ❑ Wean the child from breast or bottle by his/her first birthday.

Twelve to 24 Months of Age

- ❑ Follow the schedule of dental examinations and cleanings, as recommended by your child's pediatric dentist. Generally, dental examinations and cleanings are recommended every 6 months for children and adults.
- ❑ As your child learns to rinse his/her mouth, and as most deciduous (baby) teeth have erupted by this age, brushing with a pea-sized portion of fluoridated toothpaste becomes appropriate.

Facts about Deciduous Teeth

Proper care of a child's deciduous teeth (also known as "baby" or primary teeth) is very important as these teeth hold space for the future eruption of permanent teeth.

- ❑ If a baby tooth decays or is removed too early, the space necessary for the permanent teeth is lost and can only be regained through orthodontic treatment.
- ❑ Infected baby teeth can cause the permanent teeth to develop improperly resulting in stains, pits, and weaker teeth.

Most children begin losing their baby teeth around the age of 4 — usually the front teeth first. They continue to lose baby teeth until the age of 12 or 13 when all of the permanent teeth finally come through.

Diet and Dental Care for Children

The American Academy of Pediatric Dentistry

recommends the following to ensure your child eats correctly to maintain a healthy body and teeth:

- ❑ Ask your pediatric dentist to help you assess your child's diet.
- ❑ Shop smart. Do not routinely stock your pantry with sugary or starchy snacks. Buy "fun foods" just for special times.
- ❑ Limit the number of snack times; choose nutritious snacks.
- ❑ Provide a balanced diet, and save foods with sugar or starch for mealtimes.
- ❑ Do not put your young child to bed with a bottle of milk, formula, or juice.
- ❑ If your child chews gum or sips soda, choose those without sugar.

The Importance of Mouthguards

A mouthguard, usually a flexible piece of plastic that fits into the mouth, should be worn during all recreational and athletic activities to protect the mouth and teeth from serious injury—especially activities where there is contact or potential contact with another person, piece of equipment, or the ground. In particular, mouthguards should be worn during the following sports:

- ❑ football
- ❑ soccer
- ❑ rugby
- ❑ wrestling
- ❑ baseball
- ❑ softball
- ❑ lacrosse
- ❑ field hockey
- ❑ ice hockey
- ❑ martial arts
- ❑ boxing

Some of these sports require the use of a mouthguard at the amateur level.

Many recreational activities such as skateboarding and bicycling, also pose a risk of injuring the mouth and teeth. Exercise caution during these activities.

Mouthguards and Preventable Injuries

Injuries to the teeth, mouth, and head may include the following, many of which could be prevented with proper and consistent use of a mouthguard:

- ❑ dislodged or knocked out tooth/teeth,
- ❑ concussion,
- ❑ cerebral hemorrhage,
- ❑ broken or chipped tooth,
- ❑ bitten or lacerated tongue and/or lip,
- ❑ objects caught/lodged between the teeth,
- ❑ jaw fracture,
- ❑ neck injury, and
- ❑ jaw collision—the upper jaw gets jammed into the lower jaw.

Appendix V

FREE RADICALS AND ANTIOXIDANTS

(Universal Medicare)

We have four vital organs whose minutest affection can translate into difficulty in functioning as well as dim the chances of survival! From top to bottom, these are the brain, the two eyes, heart and the two kidneys. Any of these structures being affected can be catastrophic, and hence, it is but natural to adopt means whereby the common ailments affecting these vital structures could be warded off.

In this book, the eye is the Free Radicals and Antioxidants, "The two commonest eye problems are cataract development, and occurrence of macular degeneration, *both being aging-related*. It would be a sweet welcome for measures which holds promise in preventing cataract and aging-related macular degeneration (ARMD), so that one continues-to enjoy the same clear and sharp vision as in the younger days.

It has now been amply demonstrated that free radicals play an important damaging role in both cataract as well as ARMD. If antioxidants, *including carotenoids*, are consumed on a regular basis we have a hope of preventing these two maladies, or at least a chance of delaying the occurrence. Besides, certain carotenoids also have an additional benefit in replenishing the pigment of macula which is deficient in ARMD, and vital for crystal-clear vision.

In this Appendix the wonders of carotenoids and antioxidants for the eye especially have been put forth. These should definitely facilitate our acceptance of a new preventive approach for protecting our eyes from the aging effects.

Cataract

About 98% of the dry weight of the eye lens is proteins. The fibers in the lens are altered by unchecked free

FIG

Stages of Cataract

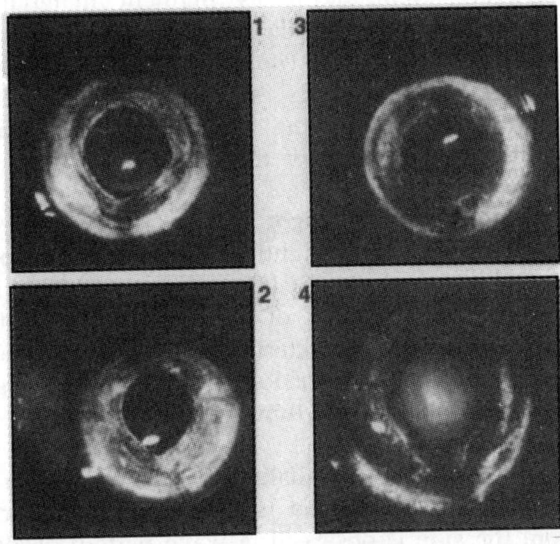

radicals rampage, leaving vision-interfering opacities known as cataracts.

Senile cataracts are the result of years of damage and accumulated oxidation. Proper levels of antioxidants, and a vital antioxidant enzyme, glutathione peroxidase, are critical for protecting the eye against cataract formation). In addition to glutathione peroxidase, even the antioxidant enzyme superoxide dismutase (SOD) activity is significantly decreased in cataractous lens.

ARMD

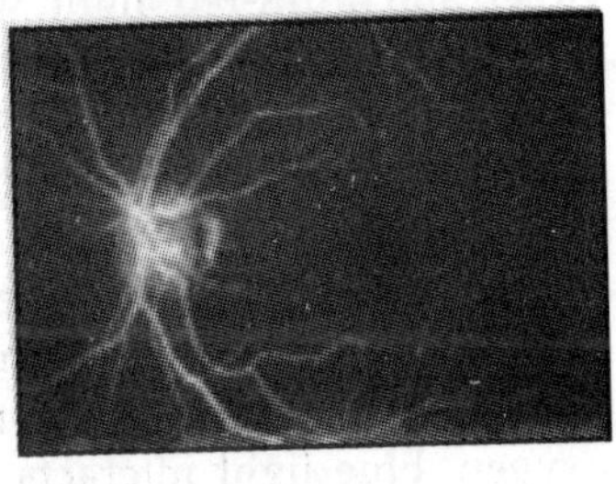

The innermost retina coat of the eye has rods and cones which facilitate conversion of light signals into electrical impulses for facilitating vision. Macula lutea, the point of maximum visual acuity, is Latin for 'yellow spot'. Macula has only cones and its central most-sensitive part is called the fovea centralis.

Lutein and zeaxanthin are two carotenoid types which are selectively accumulated as pigment material by the retina—especially the macula; this is responsible for the yellow colour of the latter. The pigment is most dense at the center fovea, and declines at the periphery. Lutein is predominant throughout the retina, whilst zeaxanthin is concentrated in the center of the macula.

Relevant Information on Light Waves

Light consists of weightless particles (that contain no mass) travelling at about 186,000 miles or 300,000 kilometers per second. These particles of light are called photons. But light also exhibits the characteristics of a wave. Wave activity is explained by imagining a long rope tied to the side of a wall and a girl shaking rhythmically one end of the rope up and down.

Each up and down shake of rope is a cycle and the number of cycles per second is the wave's frequency. If the rope from the side is observed, a wave pattern of alternating crests and troughs will be seen. The distance from one crest to another is the wavelength. As the frequency of light increases, the wavelength decreases and as the frequency decreases, the wavelength of light increases.

The frequency of light determines its colour. All the rainbow colours starting from violet to red, constitute the spectrum of light colours. Blue light has relatively the highest frequency and the shortest wavelength, whilst red light is the opposite. The eyes are sensitive to only a small part of the spectrum of frequencies, i.e. from violet to red. There is ultra-violet and infra-red light which are just beyond the eyes' range.

Ultraviolet light is filtered out by the cornea and lens in the eye, but visible blue light reaches the retina. Because the wavelength of blue light is roughly the size of an atom of oxygen, blue light interacts with the oxygen and is scattered by

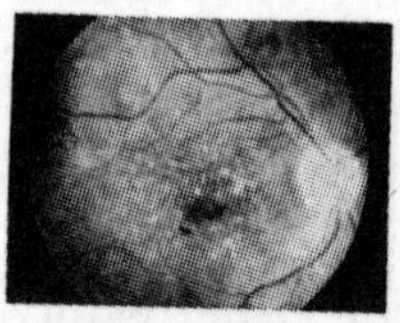

FIG

Early ARMD

it, while red light, with its longer wavelength, goes right pass the oxygen atoms. Blue light, by interacting with oxygen atoms present, generates free radicals that destroys the pigment of macula.'

ROLE OF MACULAR CAROTENOIDS

The Macula Normally Protects against the Actinic Damage:

- Passively by screening potentially harmful short-wave light due to the presence of the macular pigment.
- Actively by destroying free radicals because of the presence of lutein/zeaxanthin.

When the pigment in the macula is deficient, the latter loses its ability to absorb excess photon energy. Also the free radicals have a heyday in destroying the macula. This leads to development of ARMD over a period of time.

"The incidence of ARMD affects approximately 4-5 per cent of the population (in India) over the age of 50 years and may be affecting 19-20 per cent of people above 70 years of age."

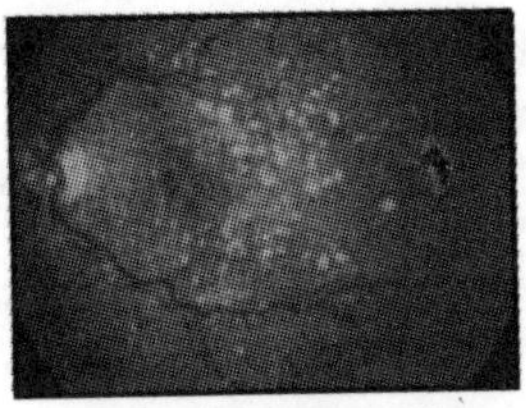

FIG

Dry ARMD

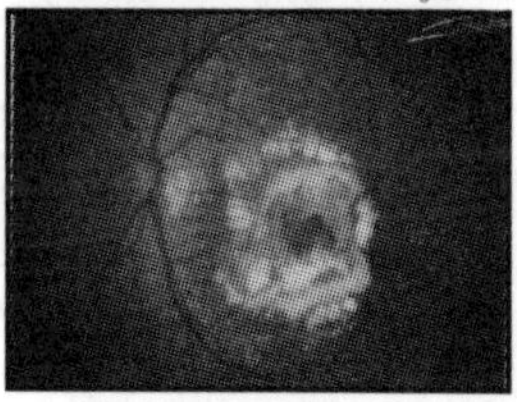

FIG

Wet ARMD

WHAT HAPPENS IN ARMD?

When the macula doesn't function well, there is blurriness or darkness in the center of any vision. Macular degeneration affects both distance and close vision and can make reading difficult or impossible.

Most patients, even those with extensive macular

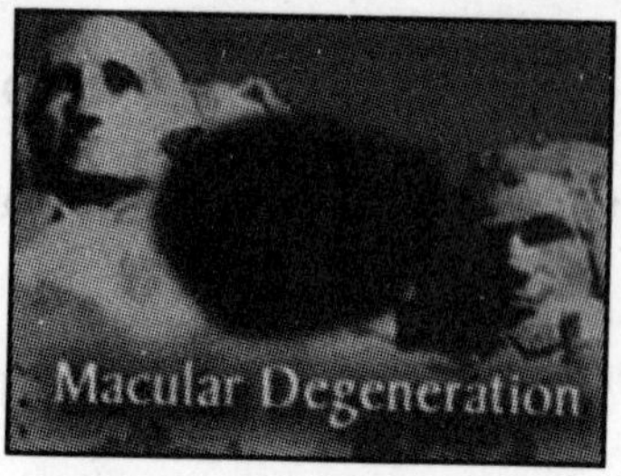

FIG.

What happens whilst seeing if there is ARMD.

involvement in both eyes, however, can maintain enough peripheral vision to walk unaided.

Patients may experience the following symptoms:

- Straight lines appear wavy,
- Colours are dim,
- Words are blurred,
- Difficulty distinguishing detail,
- Seeing flashes of light or dark spots, and
- Experiencing double vision.

Sometimes only one eye loses vision while the other eye continues to see well for many years.

REFRACTORY ERROR

Free radicals do play a role in those with myopia or shortsightedness. For those undergoing the popular laser corrective surgery for myopia (laser-assisted *in-situ* keratomileusis, LASIK; laser epithelial keratomileusis, LASEK; photorefractive keratectomy, PRK), there is always an excess generation of free radicals which can delay healing of the outer corneal surface of the eye.

FIG.

The pathway of rays of light in myopia.

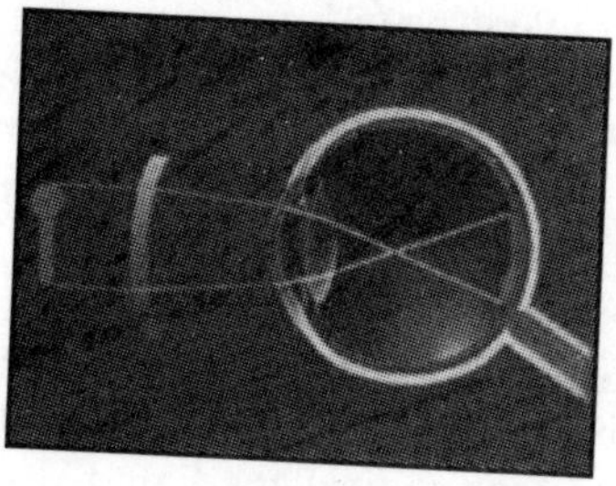

FIG.

The pathway of rays of light in hypermetropia.

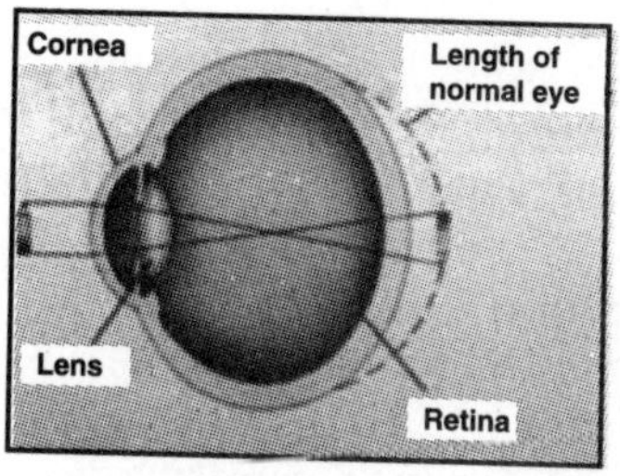

ROLE OF ANTIOXIDANTS

Replenish the Macular Carotenoids

Increased intake of these carotenoids has been shown to increase macular pigment and lower the risk of ARMD. Adequate availability of lutein/zeaxanthin in the macula protects retina from photic damage caused by the blue light. While lutein is up to 10 times more plentiful in the blood stream, the zeaxanthin which reaches the eye is preferentially drawn to the center of the macula.

Blood plasma	= 5-10 Lutein	:	1 Zeaxanthin
Retina	= 2 Lutein	:	1 Zeaxanthin
Macula	= 2 Zeaxanthin	:	1 Lutein

Protect against Free Radicals

The free radicals quickly take electrons from surrounding molecules in macula to regenerate themselves. This is fine if the surrounding molecules are some of the many antioxidants in the eye such as lutein, zeaxanthin, vitamin C or vitamin E, which are able to quench free radicals without themselves becoming free radicals. However, if these free radicals are not neutralized by antioxidants, they continue to damage surrounding molecules.

Any antioxidant supplementation must thus ensure adequate availability of all possible antioxidants which matter for the eye, if the free radical mediated damage to structures like lens and macula is to be prevented.

Carotenoids

Carotenoids comprise a number of individual ingredients:

1. Beta carotene
2. Alpha carotene
3. Lutein
4. Zeaxanthin
5. Beta cryptoxanthin
6. Lycopene
7. Other unidentified carotenoids

Carotenoids play an important role in the prevention of age-related macular degeneration, cataracts, and other blinding disorders. The best studied carotenoids are beta carotene, lutein, zeaxanthin and lycopene. Moreover, it is these three, including lycopene, which constitutes the major carotenoid content in human eye tissues, especially in the retinal pigment layer. Lycopene is an important antioxidant for protecting the lens as far as antioxidant armamentarium is concerned.

Lutein, zeaxanthin and lycopene are NOT converted to vitamin A in the body. However, lutein can be converted by body to zeaxanthin. Hence, there is never any fear of causing vitamin A toxicity.

Carotenoids are particularly effective in tackling singlet

oxygen (O_2), a reactive oxygen species (ROS) which is short-lived but has high energy and is equally very reactive and damaging like free radicals. Physical quenching involves the transfer of excitation energy from O_2 to the carotenoid, thereby producing ground-state oxygen and a carotenoid in the excited triplet state. The excess energy in the carotenoid is now dissipated as heat and the ground-state carotenoid is thus made re-available for further quenching of more O_2.

The quenching capacity of carotenoid depends primarily on the number of conjugated double bonds; lycopene has exceptionally high quenching capacity due to more number (two extra) of double bonds present in comparison to all other carotenoids.

FIG.

Chemical structure of lycopene

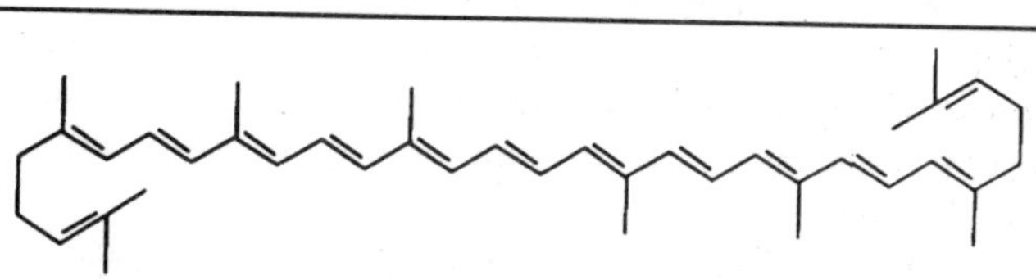

Lycopere
Mclecular Weight : 535.89
Molecular Formula: C40H56

The overall quenching capacity of alpha tocopherol is similar to beta carotene, and both are about only 1/3 that of lycopene!

Vitamins E & C

Most of the alpha-tocopherol (vitamin E) is present in the retina and choroid, and the remainder in the iris and ciliary body of the eye. The concentration of alpha-tocopherol in the eye ranges from 23 to 100 and is present at a concentration similar to other tissues, such as the liver.

Vitamin C accumulates in the ocular tissues and is one of the first antioxidants used to quench light-induced free radicals. Ascorbate also protects vitamin E from oxidation within the rod and cone cells.

Free radicals are destroyed by antioxidants such as vitamins E, C and carotenoids. The vitamins, beta carotene, E and C, plus selenium are required to allow glutathione an important antioxidant eye enzyme, to function effectively and continuously for maintaining the cellular antioxidant defenses in the war against free radicals. There is synergistic effect between vitamin E and selenium as far as antioxidant functions are concerned.

The Nutrition and Vision Project found that higher intakes of vitamin C led to a reduced risk for cortical and nuclear cataracts. Results also showed that people who used vitamin C and E supplements for more than ten years had decreased progression of nuclear cataracts.

Antioxidant Minerals

When the protective antioxidant enzyme glutathione's (especially) levels in the eye decrease, there is an accompanying increase in the light's potential to damage the macula. This results in a diminishing of vision and even in loss of vision.

Hence, *selenium* availability is vital to ensure adequacy of glutathione peroxidase antioxidant enzyme. A direct relationship exists between blood glutathione peroxidase activity and plasma selenium levels upto 100 ng/ml. Any lesser concentration means that the glutathione peroxidase activity will be submaximal.

SOD plays an important role in retinal protection against free radicals. *Zinc, manganese* and *copper* are essential for replenishing the antioxidant enzyme SOD's levels; zinc, in fact, is highly concentrated in the retina and surrounding tissues and is also an essential requirement for chemical reactions in the retina.

Copper and *zinc* are also essential for the antioxidant enzyme, catalases which has been demonstrated to be depleted in cataract.

When to Consider Antioxidants?

Many people do not realize that they have a problem until blurred vision becomes obvious. Although the ophthalmologist can detect early stages of ARMD during a medical eye examination the vision can be easily checked by using an Amsler grid.

FIG.

Amsler Grid

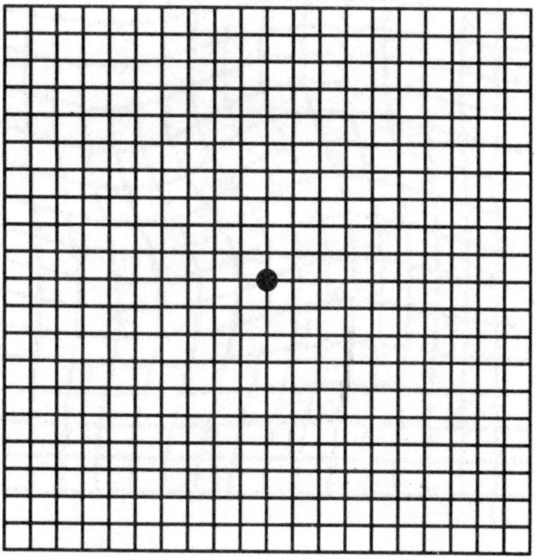

To use the grid:

1. Wear your reading glasses and hold it 12-15 inches away in good light.
2. Cover one eye.
3. Look directly at the center dot.
4. While looking at the center dot, note whether all of the lines in the grid are straight or if any lines are distorted, blurred or missing.
5. Repeat with the other eye.
6. If any lines are wavy, dark, blurred or missing, contact your ophthalmologist immediately.

Pieces of the grid disappear when an ARMD patient focuses intently on the central spot alone. To examine the grid in bright light always use the reading glasses or else the

FIG.

Amsler grid as seen in an ARMD Patient

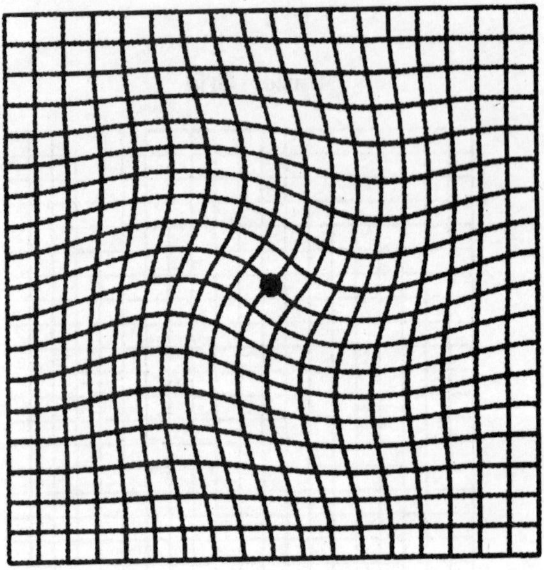

grid will seem blurry. If the lines are bent or missing vision is affected, ARMD could be the cause.

The fluid in the retina from the leaking blood vessel causes this distortion of lines, which is called metamorphopsia.

Also consider antioxidants when any of the following risk factor for ARMD is present:

- Family history of this disorder.
- Cigarette smoking.
- Low dietary intake of antioxidants.
- Female sex (macular pigment density is 0.33 + 0.15 in males and 15% lesser in females).
- Light-coloured iris.
- Presence of cardiovascular disease.
- Increased exposure to sunlight.

Efficacy of Antioxidants

An antioxidant cocktail comprising of beta carotene, vitamins E and C, zinc and copper was demonstrated (in AREDS: The Age-Related Eye Disease Study) to reduce the risk of ARMD progression by 25% in those with advanced disease affecting one eye; risk of vision loss was also reduced by approximately 19%.

FIG.

The magic of carotenoids for the macula

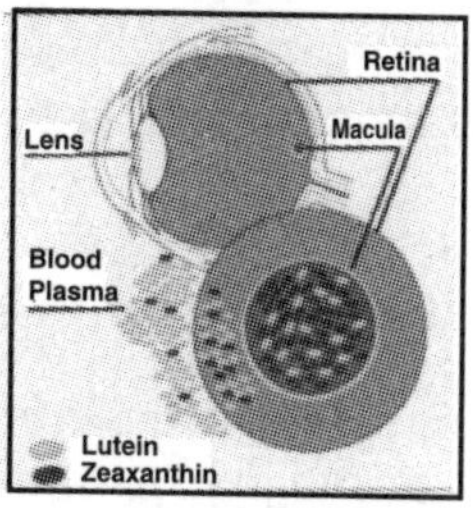

Risk factors for ARMD are:

- Low plasma carotenoids.
- Deficiency of antioxidant vitamins.
- Smoking.

Perhaps the most promising approach for the future is prophylactic treatment. Even if the rate of efficacy for prophylaxis is only 30%, such a response would still reduce by half the rate of blindness on account of ARMD.

Consuming antioxidants, particularly carotenoids, can decrease the risk of ARMD definitely. Besides, antioxidants, low-intensity laser treatment is advocated as preventive in those with risk of ARMD and having numerous large collections of a cellular, amorphous debris (drusen) in both eyes.

Requirement of Antioxidants

Beta Carotene

The requirement of vitamin A is 5,000-10,000 IU daily. 3 mg of beta carotene is equivalent to 5,000 IU of vitamin A.

Lutein

6 mg daily can increase macular pigment density significantly. Prevalence of ARMD can be reduced by half with 6 mg lutein daily.

Lycopene

The suggested requirement is 5 to 10 mg per day.

Vitamin E

3-20 mg/day is required by humans.

Vitamin C

An intake 60 mg daily permits sufficient storage of ascorbic acid.

Selenium

The recommended daily allowance (RDA) is 60-75 mcg/day; maximum safe daily intake is 450 mcg.

ZINC

RDAs are 9.5 mg for males and 7 mg in case of females. Toxicity can occur if >15 mg per day are continuously administered for prolonged periods.

Copper

Adult requirement is 0.6-0.7 mg/day; The RDA considers a safe and adequate range as 1.5-3 mg/day.

Manganese

1.4 mg/day is considered a safe intake.

Index